All-Time Favourite Animal Stories

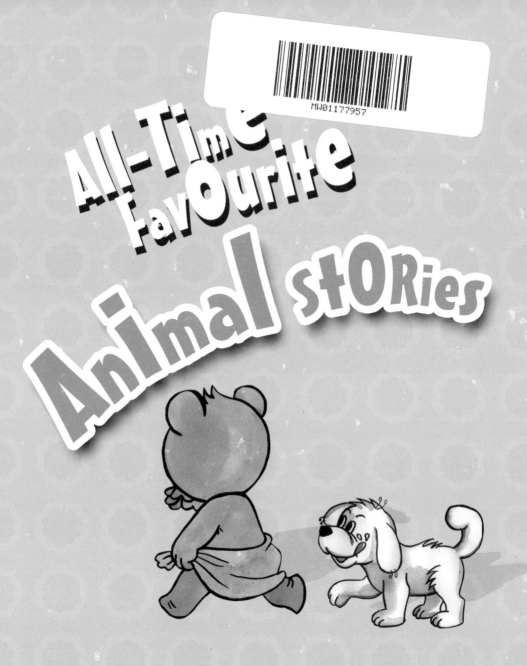

RISING SUN

Contents

Teddy Tries to Bake a Cake

One day Teddy the bear decided to bake a cake. He put all the things he needed on the table and wore his apron.

First, he put the flour and butter in a bowl. Then he broke one egg into it.

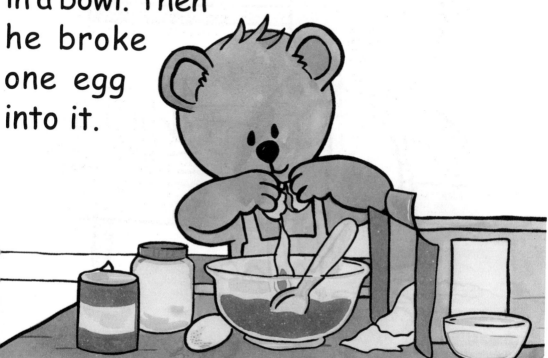

As he was breaking the other egg, it slipped from his hands. It fell on the floor and broke.

"What a mess! I will clean it later," he said to himself.

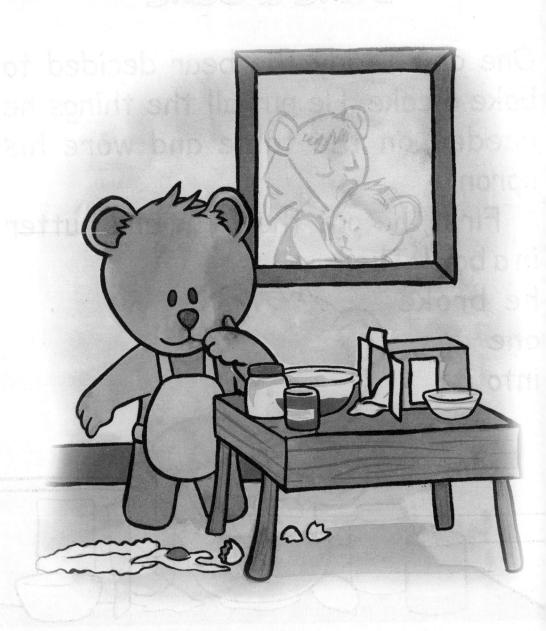

Teddy took another egg and broke it into the flour. Then he took a wooden spoon and began to mix it. After that, he added some sugar to the batter. He mixed it well. He took a spoonful and tasted it.

"Ah! This tastes good," he said to himself.

Then, Teddy added chocolate powder to it. After mixing it for a while, he tasted it again.

"Oh, it tastes better," he said, and licked his fingers.

As Teddy added each new thing to the batter, he kept tasting it till there was just a little batter left in the bowl!

Teddy put the bowl in the oven and went for a bath.

"By the time I finish my bath, the cake will be ready," he said to himself.

After his bath, when Teddy came out, he smelt something burning. "Oh, no! My cake is burning!" he cried. "What have I done!"

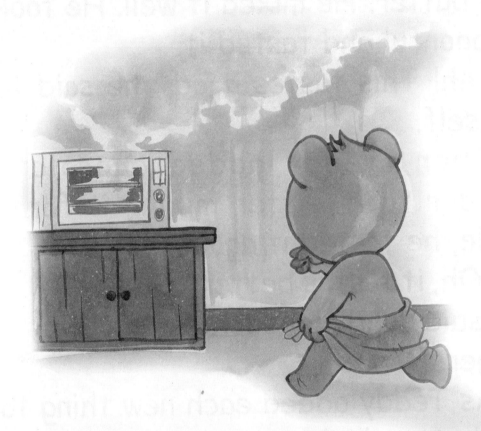

Poor Teddy had to clean up the mess and scrub the dish. And at the end of it, there was no cake to eat! Teddy was sad, but he decided to bake another cake some other day!

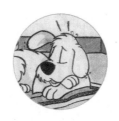

Rufus Goes For a Walk

Alan the bear lived in a small hut in the mountains. He had a dog named Rufus.

One day, Alan and Rufus were sitting by the fire.

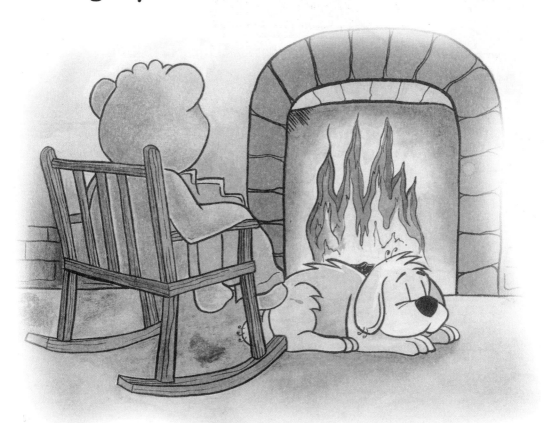

"Rufus, it's a fine day. Come on, let's go for a walk," said Alan. Rufus acted as if he was fast asleep. But Alan was not fooled by that.

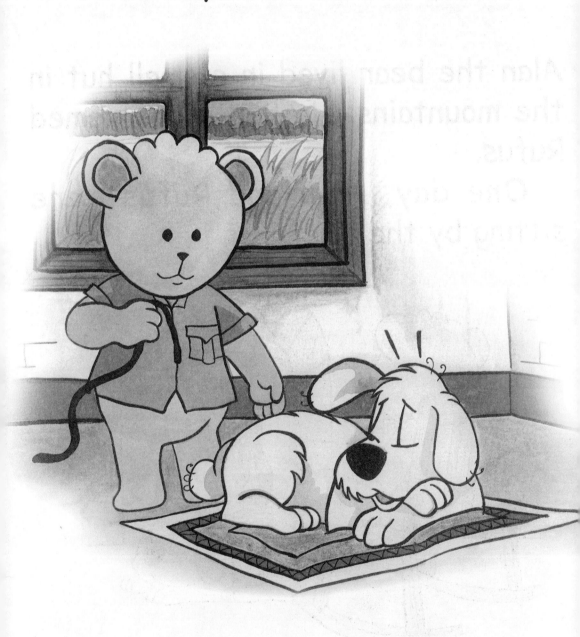

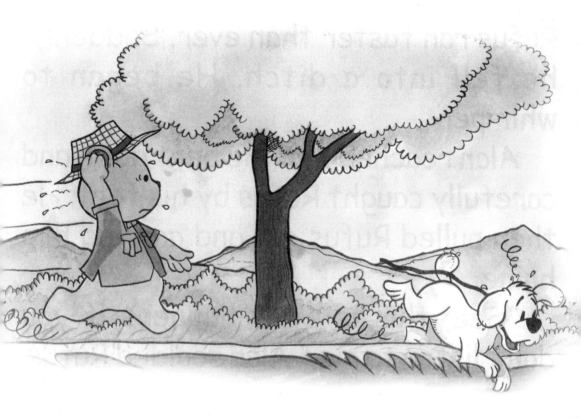

Alan fixed the leash to Rufus's collar. He then pulled Rufus out of the house and shut the door. Rufus did not want to go out as he was resting and enjoying himself. But the fresh air and the mountain flowers made him happy. He started running ahead.

"Rufus, wait. I cannot run as fast as you," said Alan. But Rufus did not listen. So Alan let go of the leash.

Rufus ran faster than ever. Suddenly, he fell into a ditch. He began to whimper.

Alan reached him. He bent down and carefully caught Rufus by his feet. He then pulled Rufus out and carried him home.

"See, this is what happens if you don't listen to me," Alan scolded Rufus.

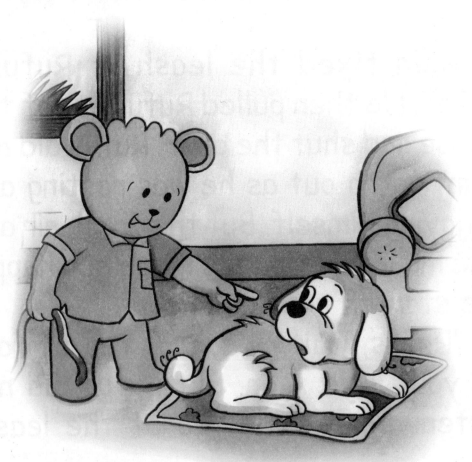

Alan bathed Rufus and then gave him some hot milk.

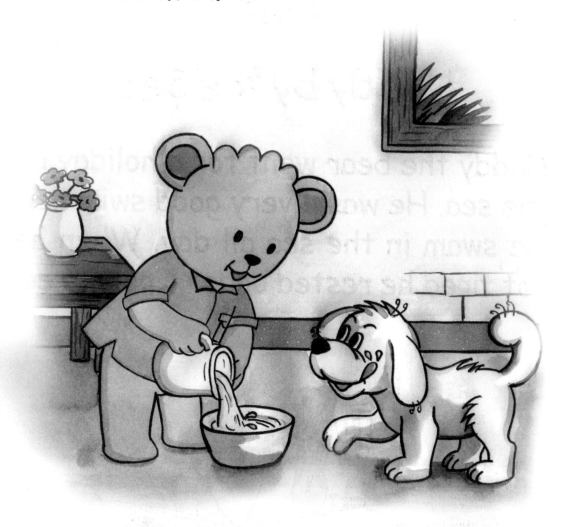

After that Alan covered Rufus and went to his rocking chair. Rufus curled up in front of the fireplace and Alan sat rocking and watching Rufus. Soon, they both fell asleep.

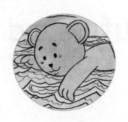

Noddy by the Sea

Noddy the bear went for a holiday by the sea. He was a very good swimmer. He swam in the sea all day. When he got tired he rested under a palm tree.

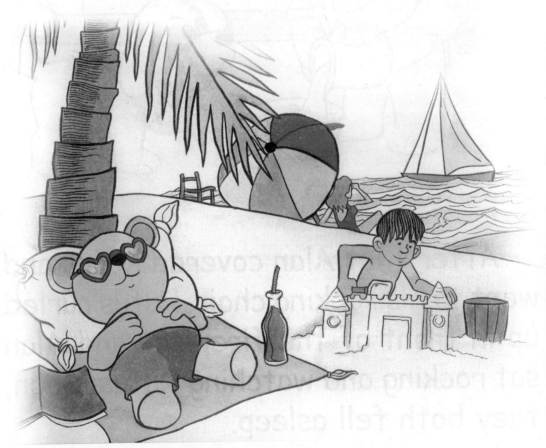

While resting, he saw some people water-skiing. "I wish I could also water-ski," he said to himself. But he did not have water-skis.

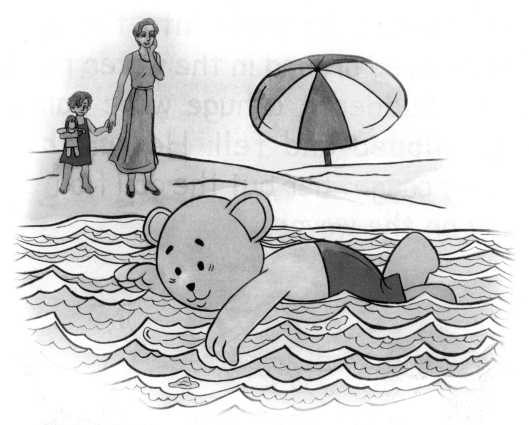

One day a young girl, Rita, came to the beach with her mother. The little girl was very pretty. She had a beautiful doll in her arms. When Noddy went to swim, they watched him.

"Mother, doesn't the bear swim well?" said Rita.

"Yes, he does," replied her mother.

After a while, Rita and her mother also decided to wade into the sea. They played around in the water for a while. Suddenly, a huge wave came. Rita slipped and fell. Her mother quickly caught her but the doll floated away on the waves.

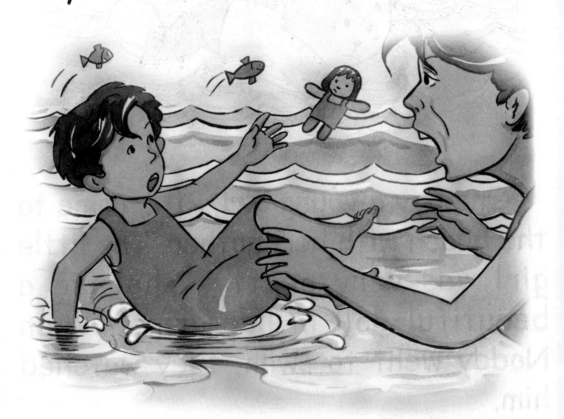

"Oh, my doll!" Rita cried. "I want my doll back."

She tried to get her doll back but her mother held on to her tightly.

When Noddy saw what had happened, he swam towards the doll as fast as he could. Soon, he was able to catch the doll. He swam back with it and gave it to Rita.

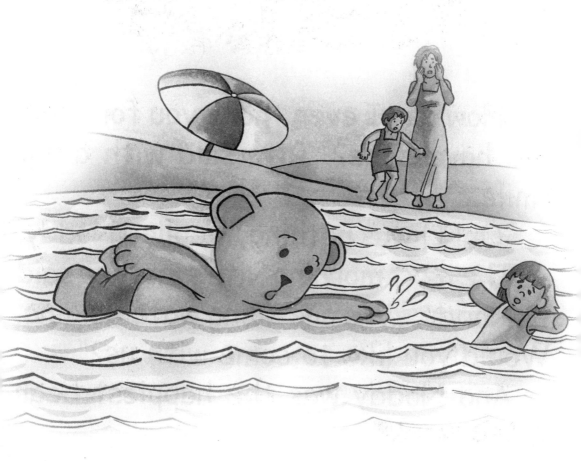

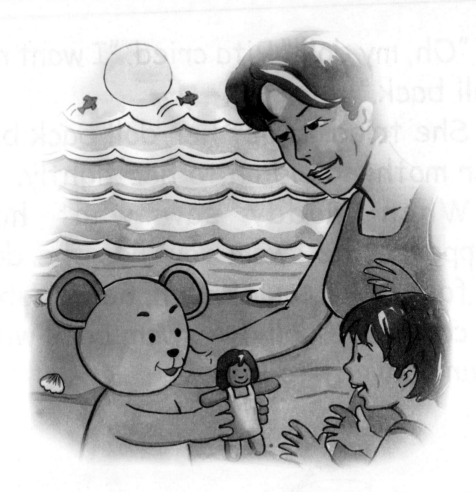

"How can I ever thank you for what you have done?" Rita said with a big smile.

"Oh! It was nothing," replied Noddy.

The next morning Rita's mother said to Noddy, "We are going water-skiing. Would you like to come with us?"

And Noddy was the happiest bear in the world!

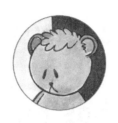

Ned's Shadow

Ned the bear loved to play outdoors all the time. He was always jumping around. He whistled and skipped all day long. But what Ned liked the most was his shadow.

He spent so much time playing with his shadow that it seemed to be his best friend.

One day, when Ned was dancing under

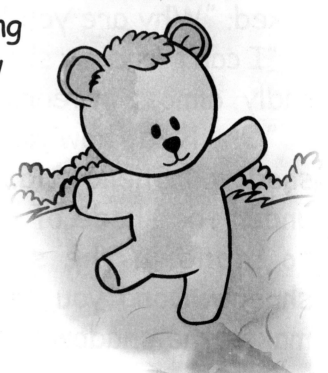

a large tree, he saw that his shadow was missing.

"Oh! Where has my shadow gone?" he wondered.

Ned looked all around. But he could not find his shadow. He missed playing with it.

Just then, a little girl called Sheila passed by. She saw Ned sitting sadly under the tree.

"What is the matter, Ned?" she asked. "Why are you looking so sad?"

"I can't find my shadow," he replied sadly, almost in tears.

"Oh, Ned, how can you find your shadow?" Sheila said. "You are sitting under the shade of a tree. You have to stand in the sun to find your shadow. Don't you know that the sun makes the shadow?"

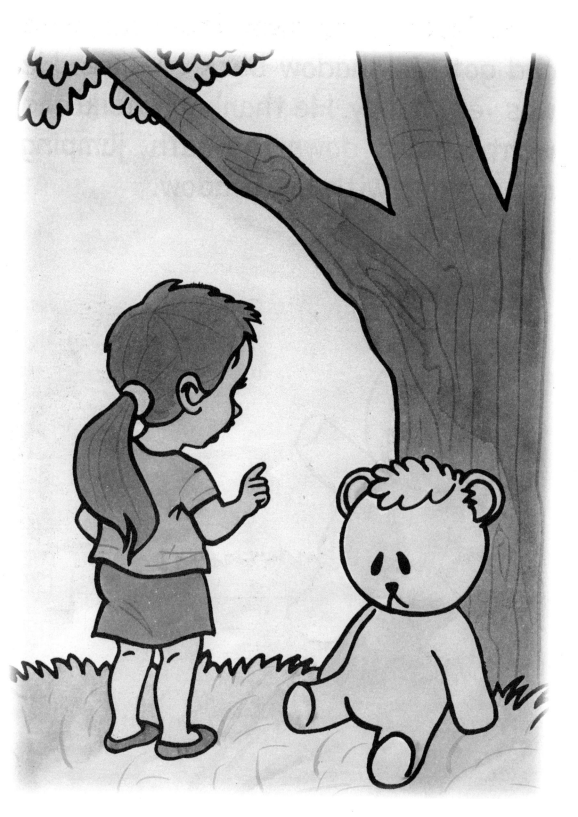

So Ned moved away from the tree and got his shadow back at once. He was very happy. He thanked Sheila and went his way down the path, jumping and playing with his shadow.

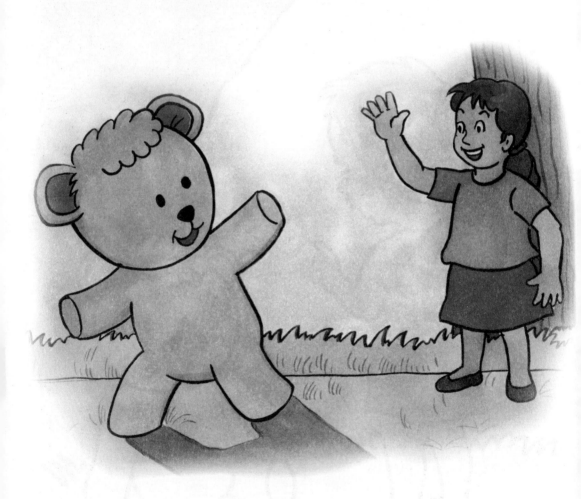

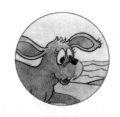

Peppy at the Beach

Peppy was a very well-behaved dog. He followed Rita, his eight-year-old mistress, everywhere. Peppy knew how to fetch the newspaper, to shake hands and to roll over. Whenever he did any of these things, Rita would give him a cola to drink. Peppy loved to make his mistress happy.

When Rita returned from school she would take Peppy to the kitchen and give him food and water. Then Rita would also have her lunch. In the evening, both Rita and Peppy would play with a ball in the lawn. Peppy loved fetching the ball. It was good fun.

One day, Peppy went to the beach with Rita. He ran here and there and rolled around on the sand. Then Rita took him near the water. But Peppy was scared. He did not know how to swim.

So Rita picked Peppy up and gently put him in the water. She held him close to her. Peppy felt safe.

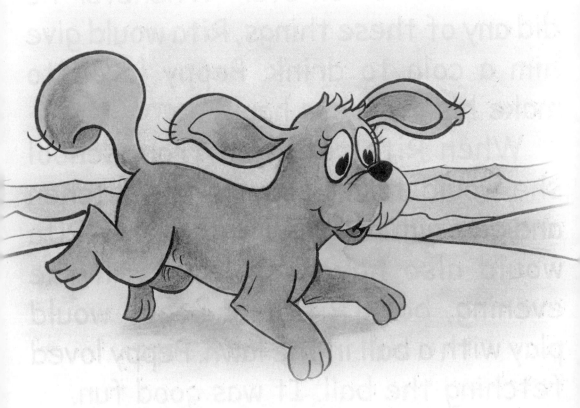

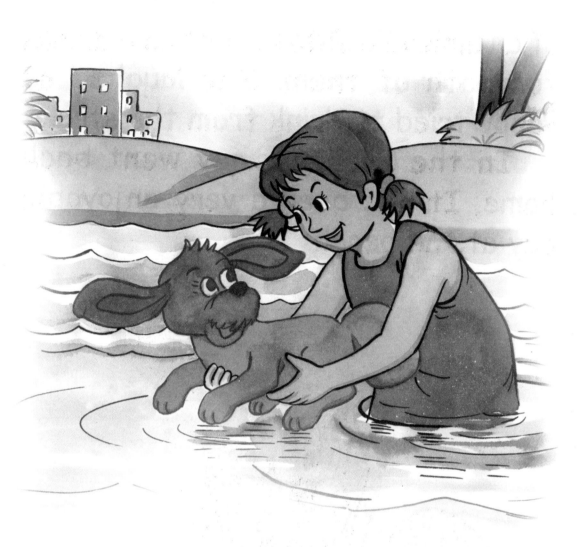

The water was nice and cool. He began to enjoy himself.

Peppy wriggled out of Rita's arms and tried to paddle. It was a lot of fun.

When Peppy got tired, they went back to the sand and sat in the shade of an umbrella. Rita bought cold drinks for both of them. She laughed as Peppy tried to drink from the straw.

In the evening they went back home. It had been a very enjoyable day at the beach.

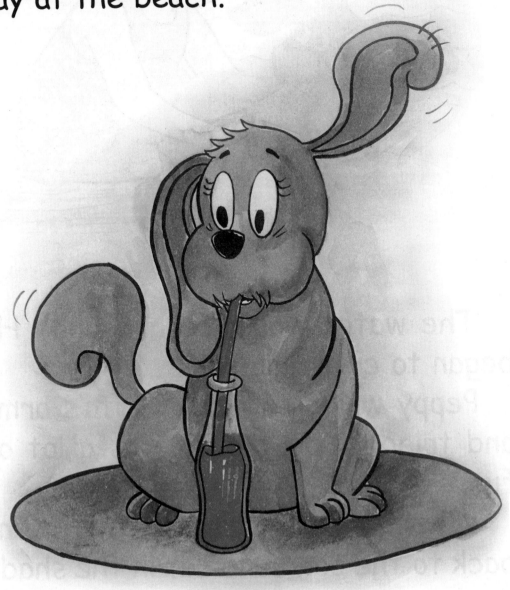

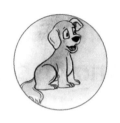

Brave Timmy

Timmy the dog lived with Michael and Jack and their parents. Mr Jacob, the children's father, ran a cafe in the front half of their house, which was near the sea.

The children loved playing on the beach. Timmy and Michael played with the ball and Jack enjoyed collecting shells.

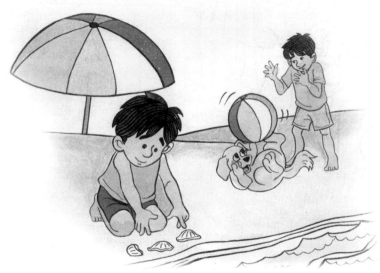

One day, Timmy and the children were busy making a sandcastle when they heard a child crying, "Mama, Mama!"

They ran towards the sea and saw a small head bobbing up and down in the water. There was no time to lose. The tide was rising fast.

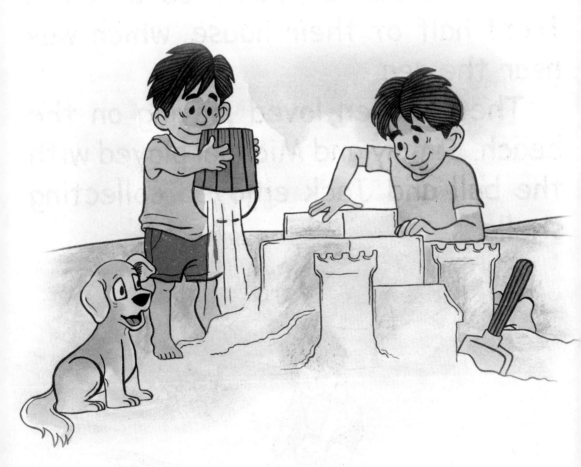

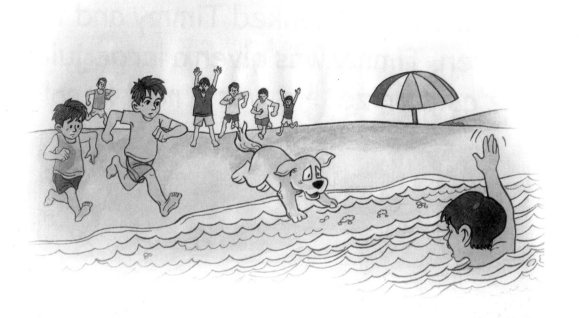

Timmy was the first to dive in. He started swimming as fast as he could. He was the first to reach the drowning boy. The boy flung his arms round Timmy's neck.

Then Michael and Jack swam up and helped the boy to get back to the shore. A group of people had collected on the beach and were waiting for them.

The parents of the boy who had been drowning thanked Timmy and the children. Timmy was given a large juicy bone as a prize. He was a real hero!

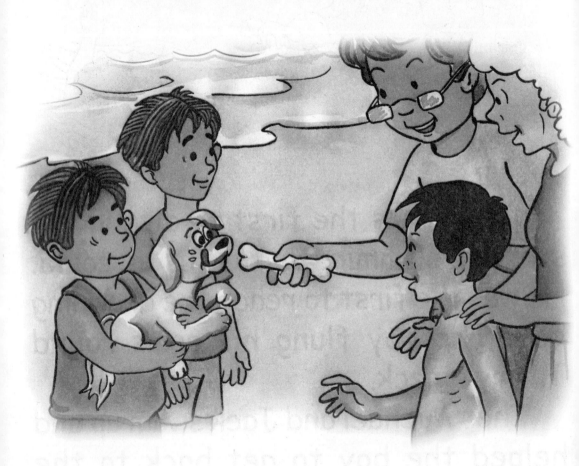

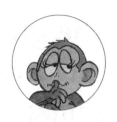

Chinky Feels Sorry

Lily lived with her parents and two elder brothers in the city.

The family was very fond of animals and birds. They had a parakeet at home.

One day, their father's friend gave them a baby monkey. The whole family

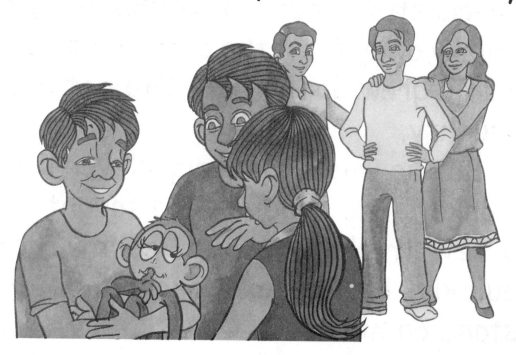

was happy with the gift. The children took turns to hold the baby monkey. After a lot of thinking they decided to name him 'Chinky'.

Chinky became part of the family. The house had a large courtyard at the back. Chinky was tied to a cot that lay there. During the winter months, the family would sit there, eating peanuts and fruits or sipping hot tea. Chinky also enjoyed the goodies.

There was one thing they all had to be careful about. They had to keep Chinky away from the parakeet's cage. As he grew up, he began to get a bit naughty.

But he was also a very clever little monkey. The children had taught him a few tricks. He had learnt them quickly. He could shake hands and stand on his head.

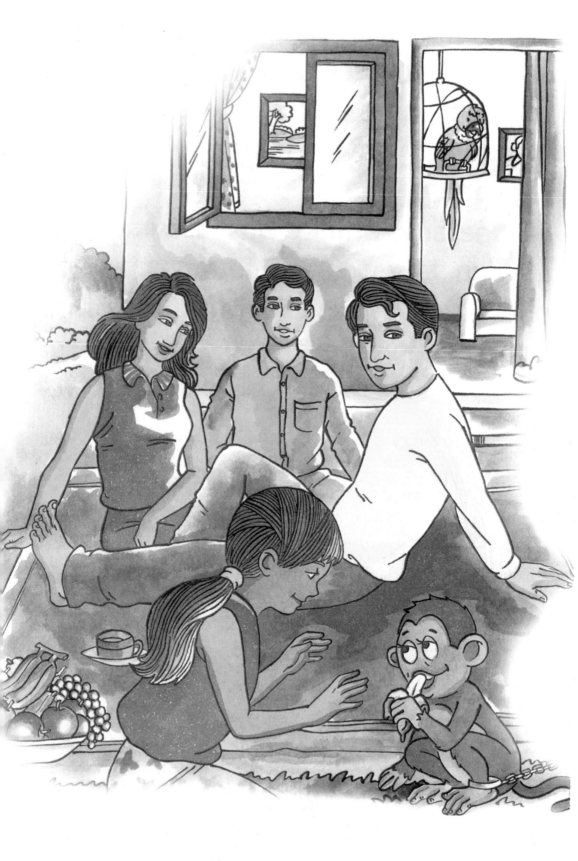

The children would take Chinky for a walk on a leash. Many people wanted to touch him. But that was not safe. He might have turned around and snapped.

One day, Chinky was playing in the garden. Lily was eating cherries while she read a book. Suddenly, Chinky jumped on her. He pulled her hair and

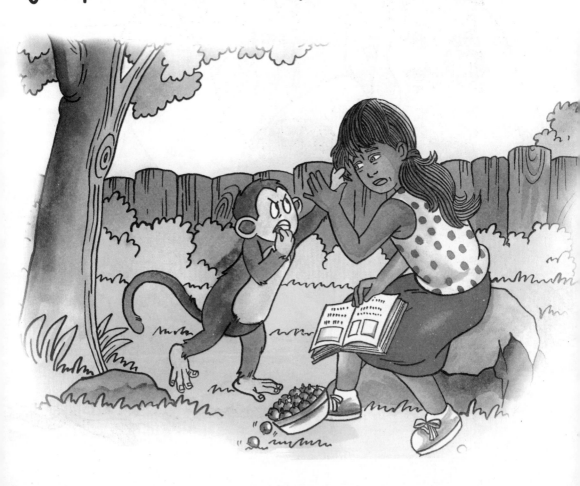

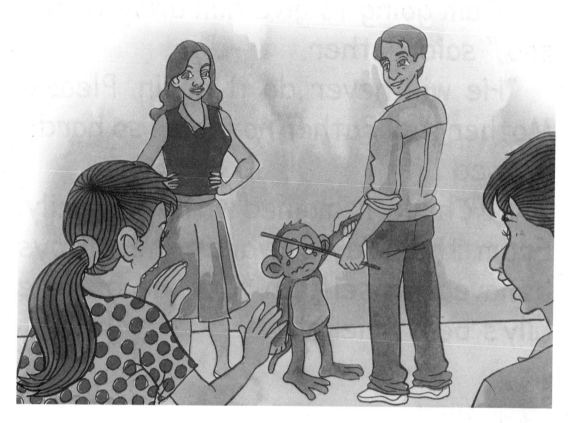

with his other paw, he started eating the cherries.

Lily screamed for help. Her family ran towards her and shooed Chinky away.

When everyone had calmed down, Chinky slowly came closer to them. He looked like he was sorry. But he had to be taught a lesson.

"I am going to give him away to the zoo," said Father.

"He will never do it again. Please, Mother, tell Father not to be so hard," begged Lily.

So Chinky remained with the family. From that day onwards, he always behaved himself. In fact, he became Lily's best friend!

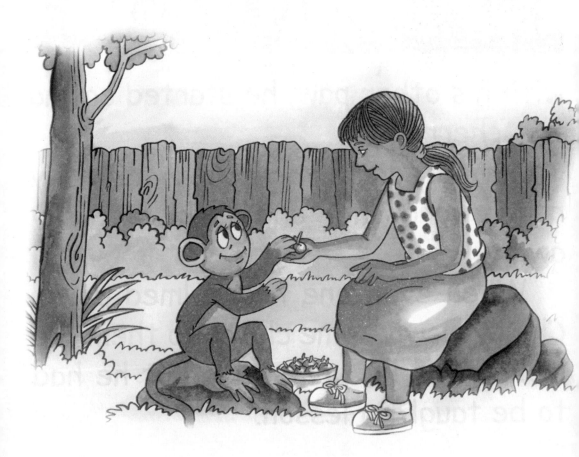

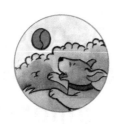

Sandy Goes to the Park

Sandy the dog loved playing with his little master, Benny. They went to the park every evening. Many other children also played there.

Sandy and Benny enjoyed playing games with the ball. Benny would throw the ball and Sandy would fetch it. He had become very good at this game.

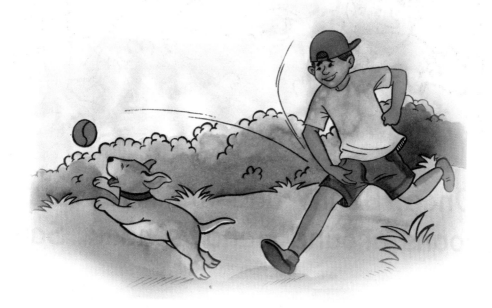

Benny's friends also joined them in their games. Sometimes they played hide-and-seek among the bushes. Sandy loved this game. When the other boys could not find Benny, they would ask Sandy to find his master. He would at once show them where Benny was hiding!

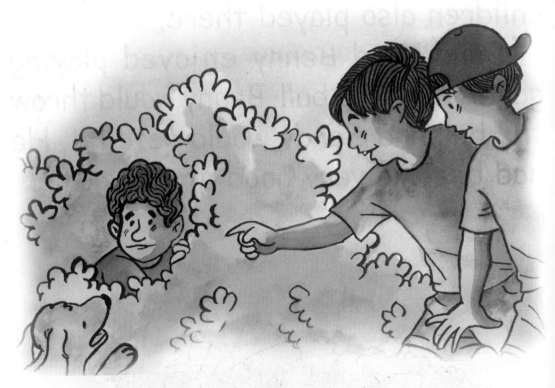

Once, Benny and his friends tied balloons around Sandy's neck. Sandy ran all around the park. The boys chased Sandy but he was too fast for them. Suddenly, the balloons burst as he brushed past a thorny bush. Sandy got scared and started barking. Benny picked him up and said, "Hush, Sandy, it's all right. Don't be scared."

One day, while the boys were playing in the park, Sandy began chasing a butterfly. He ran after it, but the butterfly flew away. Just then a man dressed in torn and dirty clothes came and caught Sandy.

The man was about to put Sandy in a bag, but the clever dog started barking loudly. The man tried to shut Sandy's mouth but Sandy bit the man's hand.

"Ouch!" shouted the man, and let Sandy go.

The boys heard Sandy bark. They ran towards the man. They tried to catch him, but he ran away.

"Never mind," said Benny. "Sandy is safe and sound."

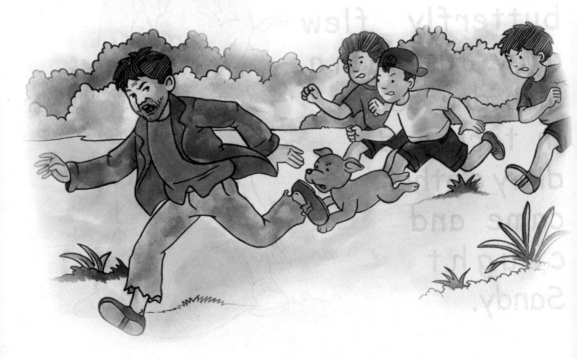

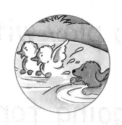

Inca Goes on an Outing

Inca, Robin's pet dog, was beautiful and golden in colour. He had come to live with Robin when he was a tiny little puppy. Now he was grown up.

Inca knew a lot of tricks. He could fetch a newspaper and shake hands.

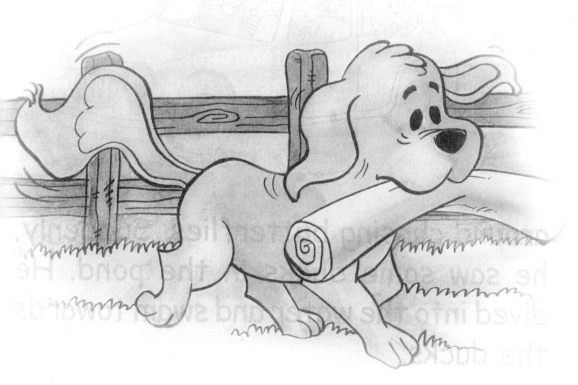

And he liked to play with a ball in the garden.

Inca loved going for a ride in the car. He barked happily when the wind blew on his face as he looked out of the window.

One day, Robin and his parents took Inca to the park. Robin took off Inca's leash and let him go free. Inca ran

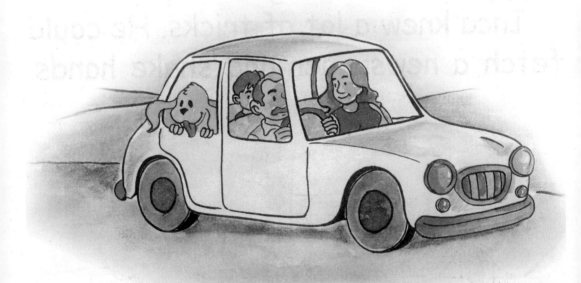

around chasing butterflies. Suddenly, he saw some ducks in the pond. He dived into the water and swam towards the ducks.

"No, Inca," shouted Robin, and ran after him.

One of the gardeners got into the water and caught Inca. The ducks were saved!

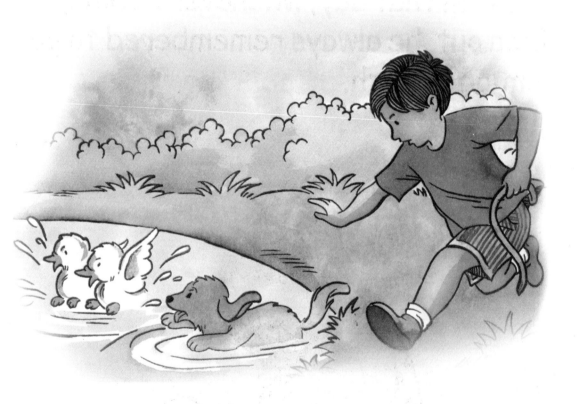

"Bad dog, Inca," scolded Robin.
Inca hung his head sadly.
They went back to the car quickly.
When they reached home, Mother

quickly dried Inca so that he would not catch a cold. Then Robin's sister Jean gave him some warm milk to drink and covered him up with a rug. Soon Inca was fast asleep.

From that day, whenever Robin took Inca out, he always remembered to put him on a leash.

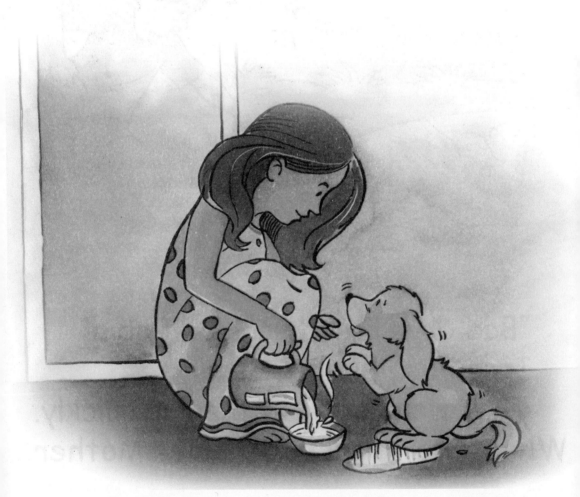

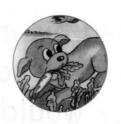

Kenny and His Master

Kenny was a beautiful dog. He had light brown hair and bright eyes. He would follow Vicky, his eight-year-old master, everywhere.

Vicky would take him for long walks and play ball with him in the garden. He also taught Kenny to jump over a stick.

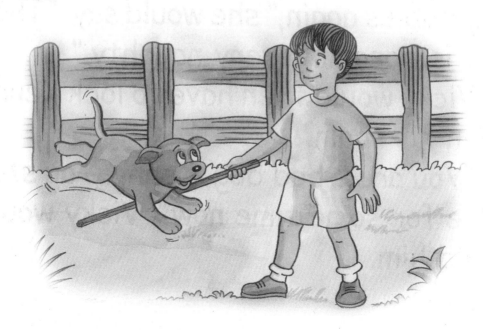

Kenny guarded his master well. No one could enter the room if Vicky was sleeping. Kenny would lie under his master's bed. If anyone tried to enter the room, Kenny's growl would stop that person. He would let people in only when Vicky woke up.

Kenny loved to dig out moles in the kitchen garden and chase them. Sometimes, he also dug out the vegetables! This made Vicky's mother very angry.

"Vicky, Kenny has dug out the vegetables again," she would say. "That dog is becoming very naughty."

Vicky would then have to lock Kenny up in his room.

"You are a bad dog, Kenny. You stay here for some time now," Vicky would scold him.

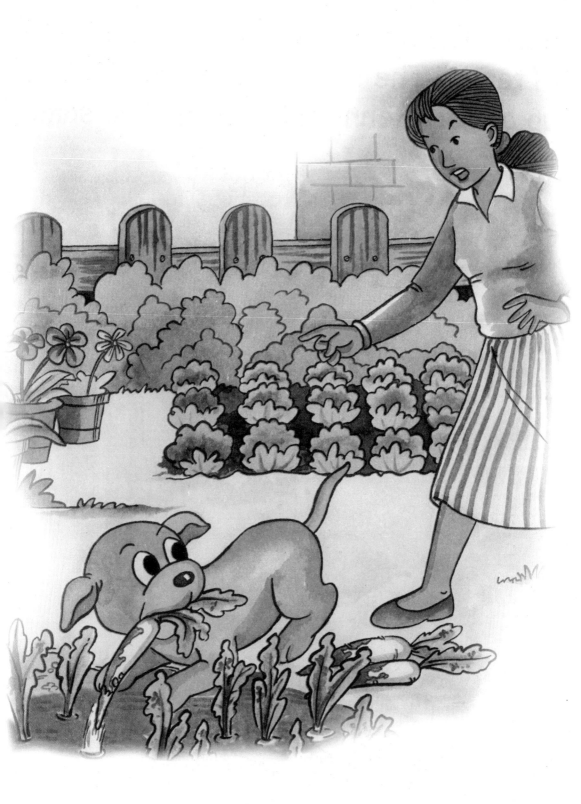

Once Kenny and Vicky went for a walk. Kenny saw a squirrel and ran after it. The scared squirrel climbed up a tree. Kenny tried to do the same

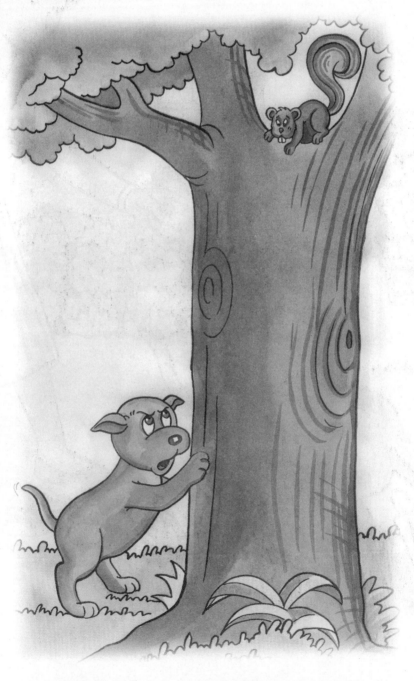

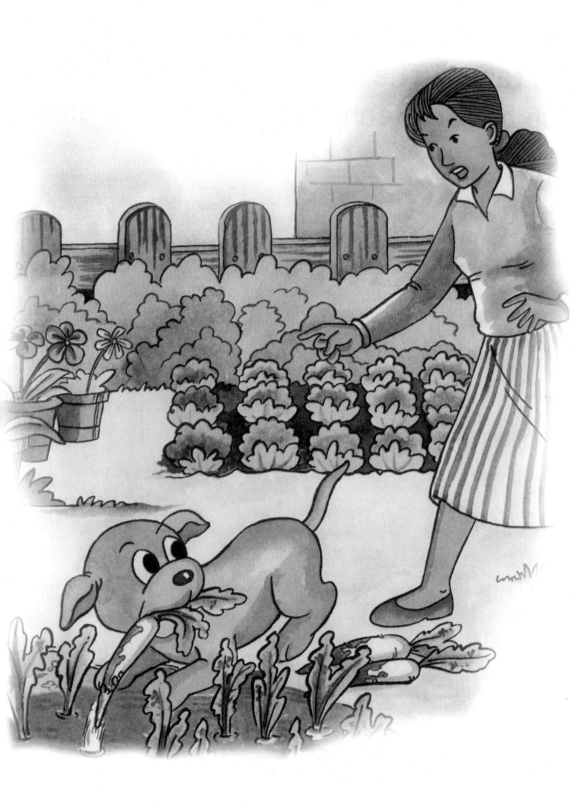

Once Kenny and Vicky went for a walk. Kenny saw a squirrel and ran after it. The scared squirrel climbed up a tree. Kenny tried to do the same

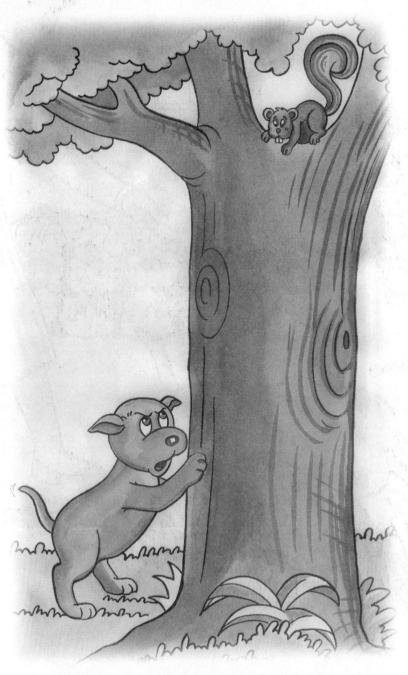

but couldn't. He started barking angrily. Vicky laughed and said, "Kenny, you're a dog, not a monkey. You can't climb trees! Come along, now."

When Vicky and his friends played cricket, Kenny would run away with the ball. So Vicky would tie him up while playing cricket. But naughty Kenny would bark till he was set free!

One day, Vicky's friend Ray decided to hide in the bushes and frighten Vicky. When Vicky and Kenny came

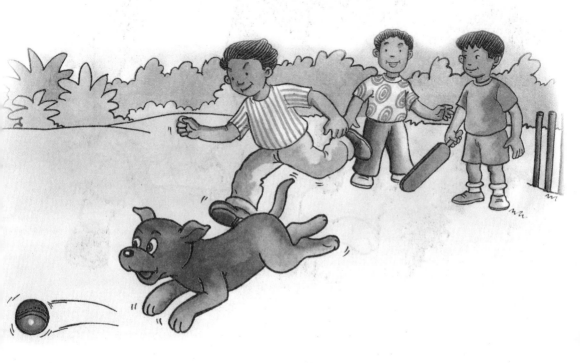

home from the park, Kenny ran straight to the bushes and began barking. Ray came out and said, "Vicky, your dog is really too clever. He won't even let me surprise you."

Vicky laughed and hugged Kenny.

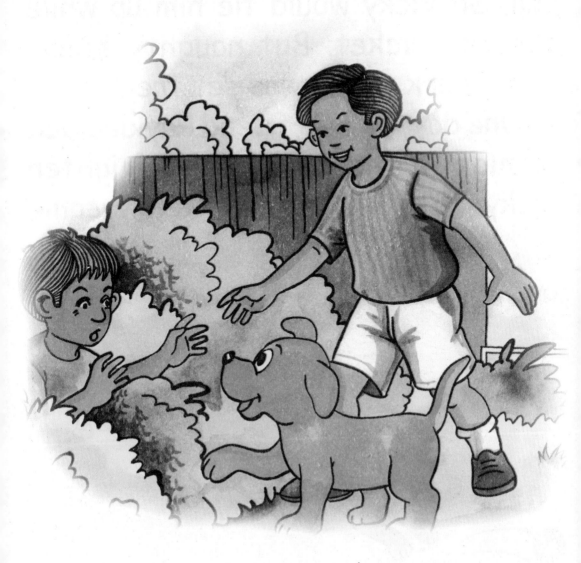

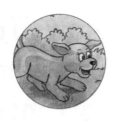

Jackie Chases a Kitten

Jackie was a clever dog. He was very fond of the family he lived with. But he did not like the two little kittens who also lived in the house. Their mewing made him angry. Henry, his master, loved the kittens, and this made Jackie even more angry.

One day, while Jackie was napping on the verandah, he heard one of the kittens mewing. He was angry and ran down the garden path to chase the kitten away.

The kitten saw Jackie rushing towards her. She jumped over the fence. Jackie hit his nose on the wooden fence. He cried out in pain.

Henry came rushing out. He lifted Jackie up and took him in to rub an ice-cube on his nose. Jackie felt better after that.

The next day, Henry took the kitten and a small ball and went to Jackie.

"Kitty wants to play with you," said Henry gently. He threw the ball and Kitty ran to catch it. She brought it back to Jackie, who pushed the ball away. Kitty mewed happily and ran to fetch it again. Slowly they began to play together.

The other kitten was watching Jackie from the branch of a tree. She was scared of him. But when she saw

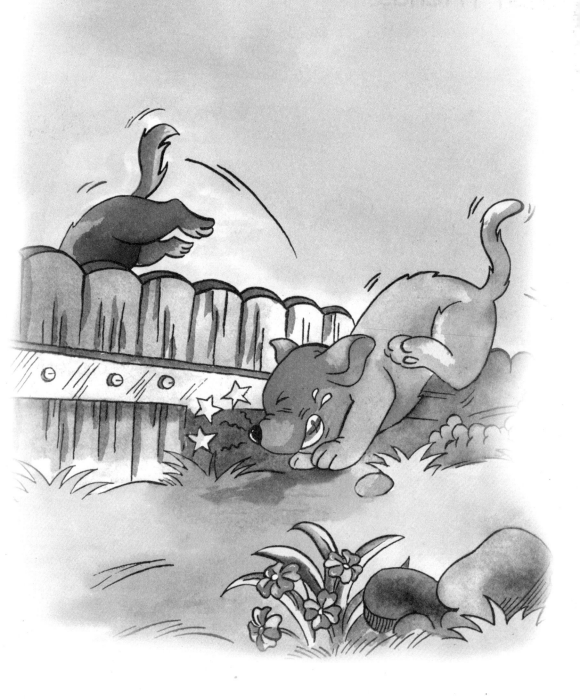

Kitty playing with Jackie, she slowly came down the tree and joined them.
Now all three of them have become best friends.

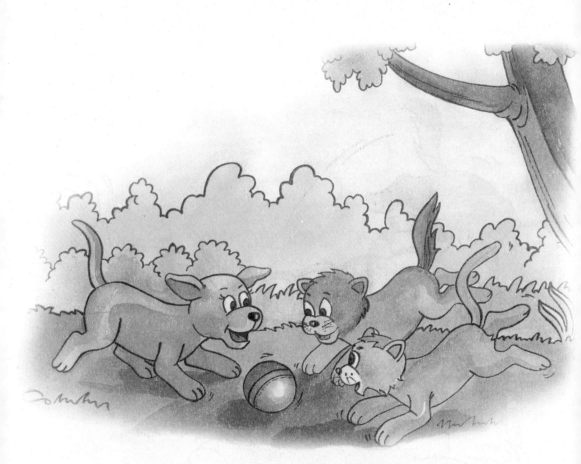

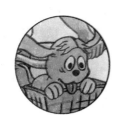

Frisky Gets a New Master

A pup named Frisky lived on a farm. He loved chasing butterflies and rabbits and squirrels. He slept in a little kennel.

Every day, a boy named Rikki from the next farm visited him.

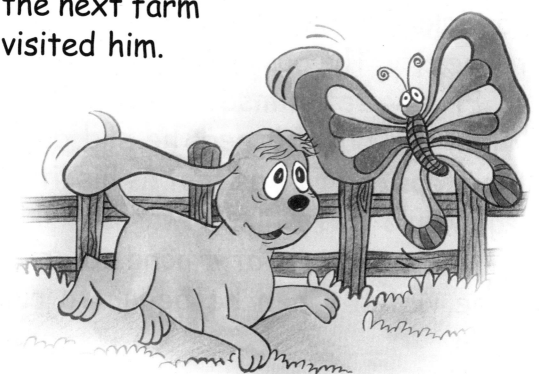

He would bring with him a biscuit or a rusk for Frisky. They were good friends.

Once, Frisky decided to visit Rikki. So he crept across to the next farm. Rikki shouted with joy when he saw the pup. He decided to give him a ride on his bicycle. Away they went, with the wind blowing on their faces. It was great fun. Frisky loved it.

One day, Ronnie, Frisky's master, was taking Frisky in a basket on a bus to the city. The basket was not locked, so Frisky set himself free easily. When the bus stopped, he slid down the steps and ran, as fast as his little legs would carry him, towards Rikki's farm. He stopped at a pond to drink some water. Then he began to run again.

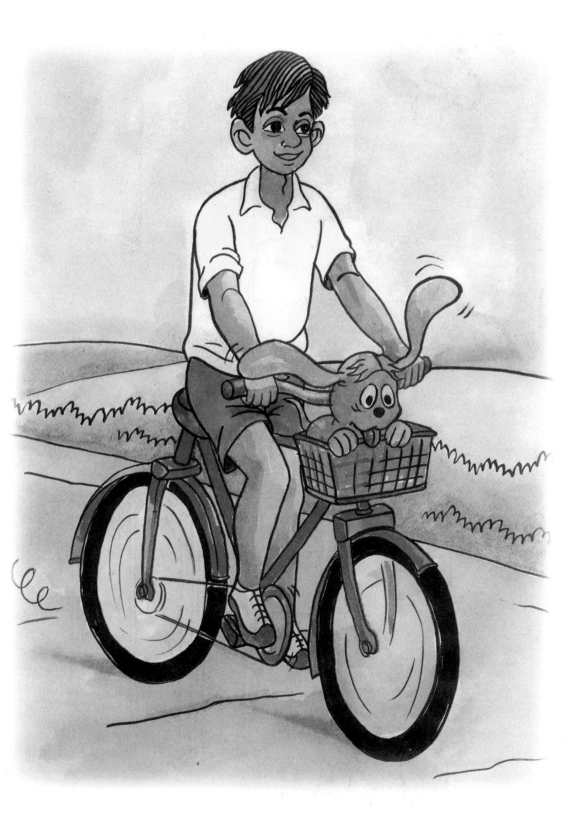

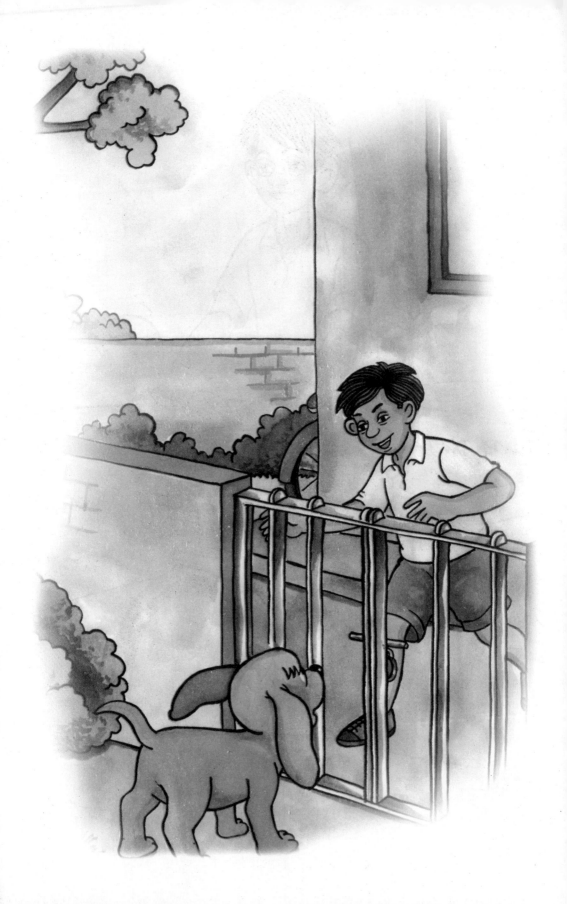

At Rikki's gate he began barking. Rikki rushed out of his house. He took Frisky in his arms and gave him a big hug. When Ronnie came home, he saw Rikki waiting for him with Frisky in his arms. Ronnie couldn't help smiling at them both.

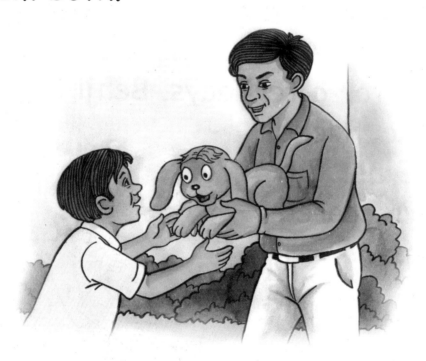

He said, "Since you love Frisky so much, and Frisky loves you too, I think I shall give him to you as a gift."

Frisky and Rikki were very happy and jumped with joy.

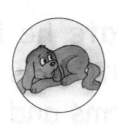

Benji Makes a Friend

Benji the dog lived with his little master Abel in a house by a beach.

One day Abel's cousin Gina came visiting for a few days. Benji wanted to make friends with Gina. But Gina was scared of dogs.

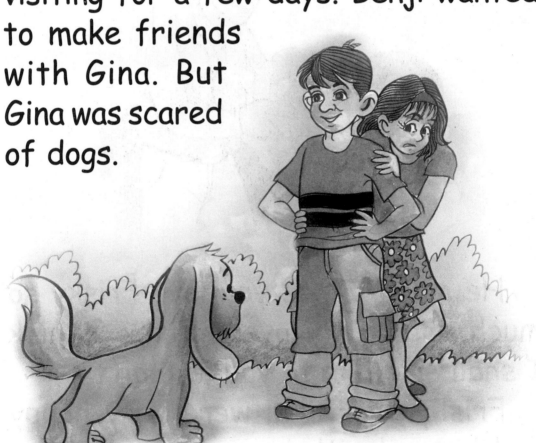

Gina only liked to play with her doll Sherry. This made Benji very unhappy and he sat sadly on the rug with his tail turned in.

One day all of them went to the beach. Poor Benji had to sit far away. He missed playing with his master. But Abel wanted to play with Gina. She had come only for a few days.

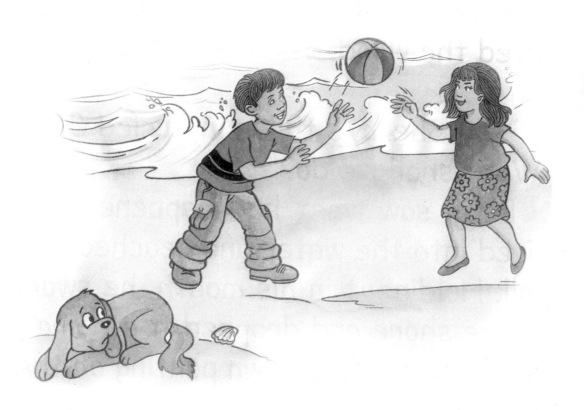

Gina saw a piece of wood floating on the waves.

" Let's give Sherry a ride," she said.

She reached out for the piece of wood, knelt down and placed the doll on it. Abel stood next to her and watched. Gina gently pushed the piece of wood and clapped her hands as it floated away on the waves.

After a while, a large wave came and tilted the wood. The doll fell into the water.

"Oh! Sherry's fallen in," cried Gina. "What shall we do?"

Benji saw what had happened. He dived into the water and reached the doll. Holding it in his mouth, he swam to the shore and dropped it at Gina's feet. Then he lay down panting on the ground.

Gina only liked to play with her doll Sherry. This made Benji very unhappy and he sat sadly on the rug with his tail turned in.

One day all of them went to the beach. Poor Benji had to sit far away. He missed playing with his master. But Abel wanted to play with Gina. She had come only for a few days.

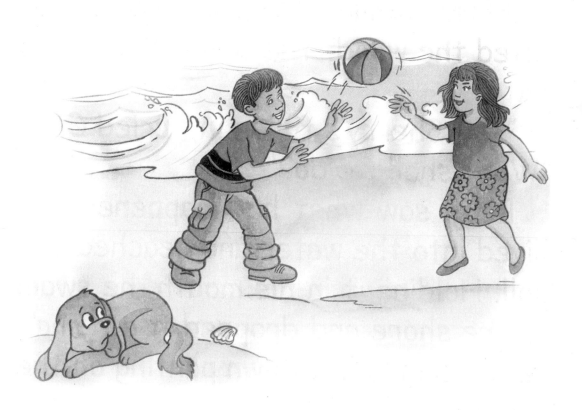

Gina saw a piece of wood floating on the waves.

" Let's give Sherry a ride," she said.

She reached out for the piece of wood, knelt down and placed the doll on it. Abel stood next to her and watched. Gina gently pushed the piece of wood and clapped her hands as it floated away on the waves.

After a while, a large wave came and tilted the wood. The doll fell into the water.

"Oh! Sherry's fallen in," cried Gina. "What shall we do?"

Benji saw what had happened. He dived into the water and reached the doll. Holding it in his mouth, he swam to the shore and dropped it at Gina's feet. Then he lay down panting on the ground.

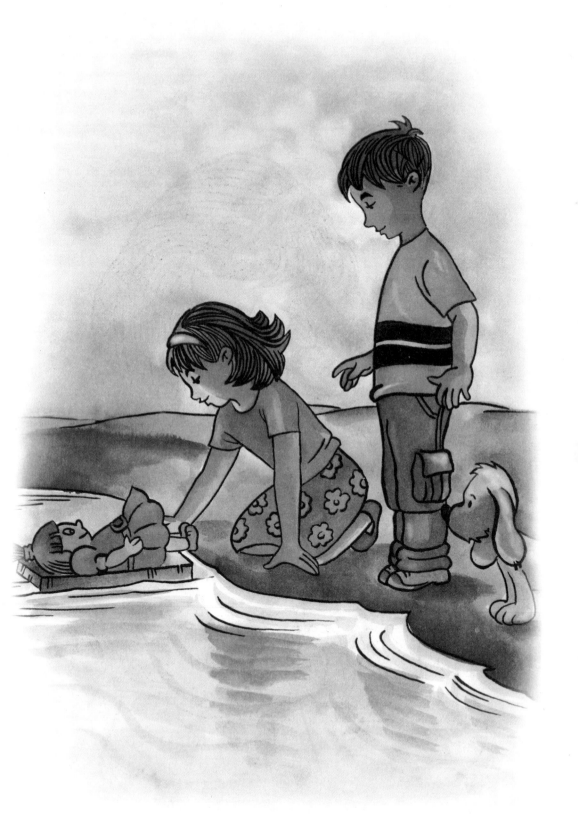

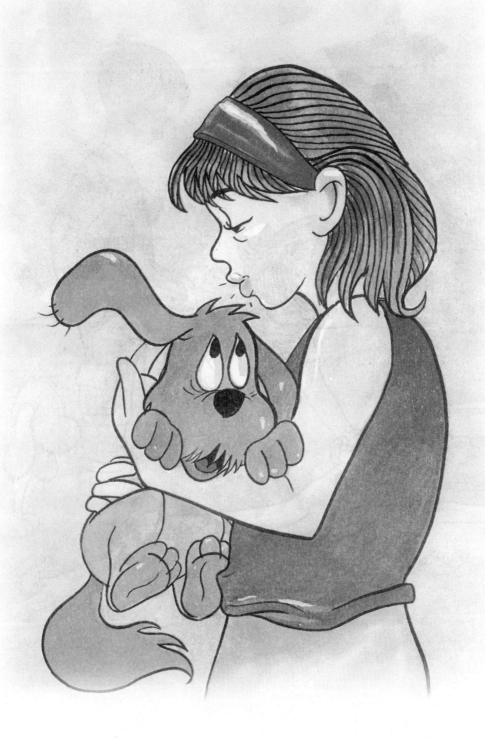

Gina lifted Benji and kissed him on his forehead.

"Thank you, Benji, for saving Sherry. I want to be your friend," she said.

Benji was very happy to hear that. He held out his paw to shake hands with Gina.

Gina was no longer scared of dogs. Now Benji did not have to sit away from the two children.

Whenever Gina played with her doll she called Benji to play too! And when Abel and Gina played with the ball, Benji also played with them.

Soon it was time for Gina to go back home. Benji was very sad. Gina kissed him goodbye and said, "I'll be back soon, Benji, I promise."

Benji wagged his tail happily.

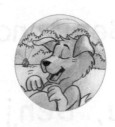

Naughty Terry

A naughty little dog named Terry lived in a house with his mother and two brothers. Whenever he was hungry, he would climb up on the kitchen stool and get onto the table. He would always find something nice to eat there.

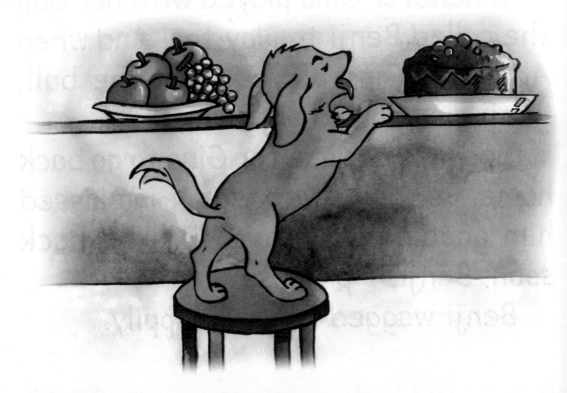

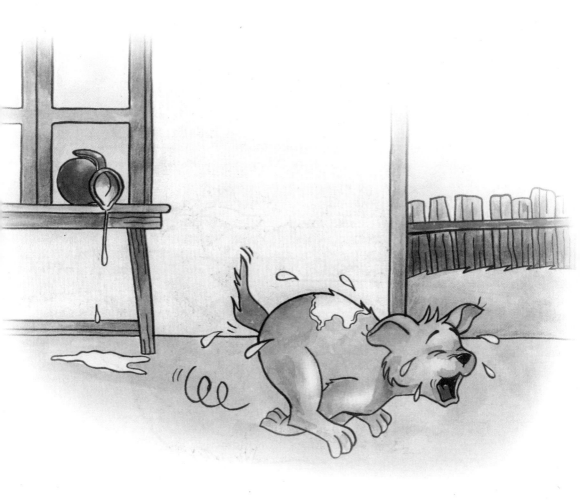

One day Terry found a big slice of chocolate cake on the table and started eating it. There was also a jug full of hot milk next to the cake. He put his head in to drink some, but the jug tilted over. The hot milk burnt his skin. He yelped and dashed out into the garden.

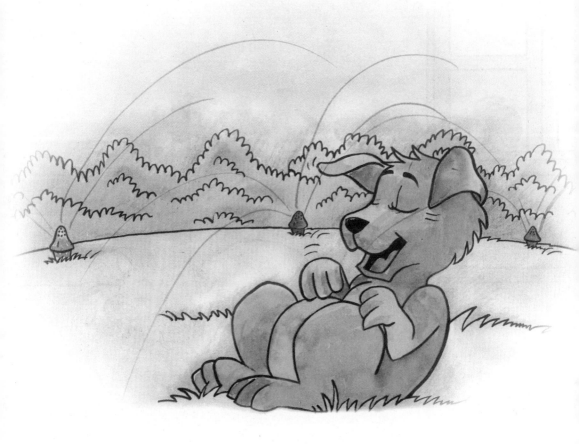

Terry saw the sprinklers spraying water on the grass. He sat on the grass and let the water cool his burning skin. Then he dried himself in the sun and went back into the house. He lay down with his family and was soon fast asleep.

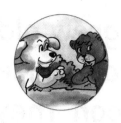

How the Dog and the Cat Became Enemies

Once there was a man, his wife and their pets, a dog and a cat. They all lived very happily together.

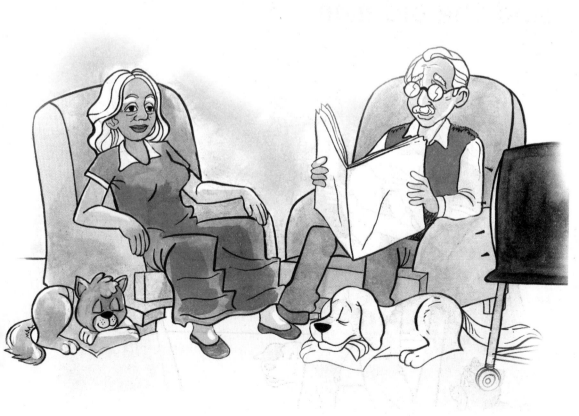

As the man grew older, he became weaker and weaker. He could not get work easily. Soon they did not have any money left. His wife had to sell her jewellery to buy food. Among the things she sold was a gold ring.

One day, they met a man who told them that they would become rich again if they got back the gold ring.

"We must get that gold ring back," said the old man.

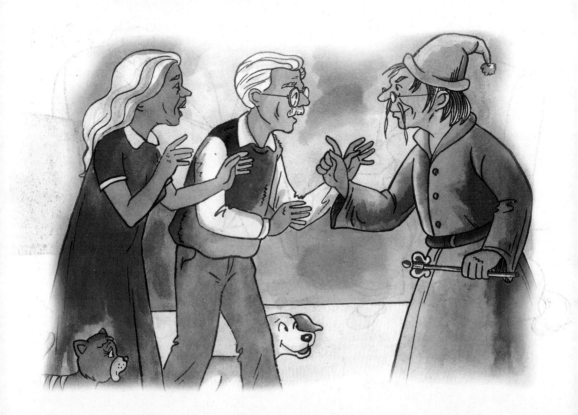

"But how can we do that?" asked his wife. "The ring is in a bag in the jeweller's house."

The dog and the cat heard these words.

"We have to get the ring back from the jeweller's bag," said the dog.

He thought of a clever plan.

"You catch a mouse and make him chew into the bag and get the ring out," he told the cat. "Tell him that you'll eat him up if he does not obey."

Soon, the cat caught a mouse. Holding him

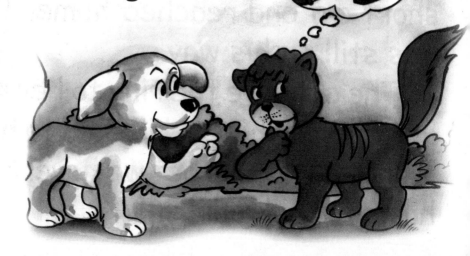

between her teeth, the cat went to the jeweller's house. The dog followed her. The mouse chewed a hole in the bag and got out the ring. He dropped the ring at the cat's feet and ran away before she changed her mind and ate him up!

The cat picked up the ring, took a short cut and reached home. The dog was still on his way.

The cat gave the ring to her master. He was very happy. He said to his wife, "What a faithful pet we have! See, she has got back our ring."

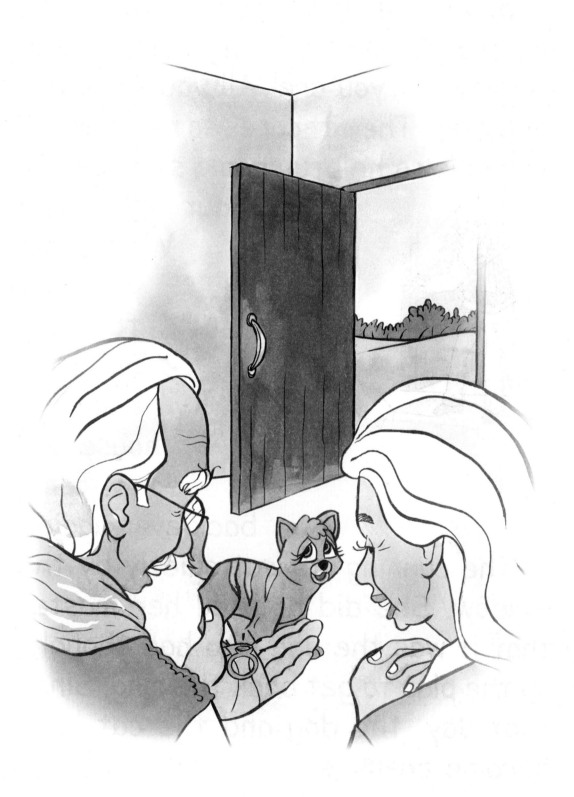

When the dog reached home, the old man scolded him angrily. "What a useless pet you are! All you do is eat and sleep. The cat cares so much about us and is so helpful. Look, she has got

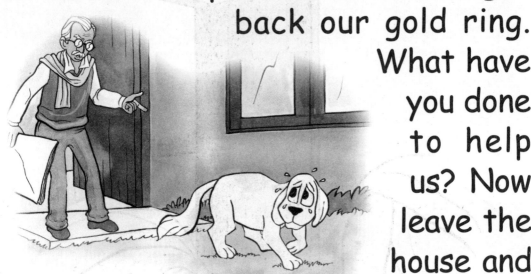

back our gold ring. What have you done to help us? Now leave the house and don't come back ever again."

The cunning cat sat quietly by the window. She did not tell her master that it was the dog who had thought up the plan to get back the ring. Since that day, the dog and the cat have become enemies.

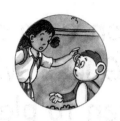

Chipsie the Monkey

Chipsie the monkey wondered why she could not go along with Ann to her school. Ann would never allow her to go with her on the bus.

Every afternoon Chipsie would wait at the bus stop for Ann to return. Ann would get down and give a big warm hug to Chipsie before telling her all the things that had happened at school that day.

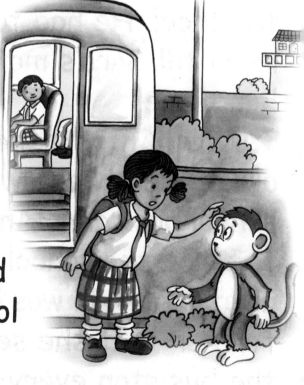

One afternoon, Ann came home and told Chipsie, "Guess what, Chipsie! I have been chosen to play in the school band. My best friend Sara is coming home so that we can practise together. She is going to sing while I play the guitar."

Chipsie liked talking to Sara, who loved pets. She had a dog named Woof. She told Chipsie that one day Woof had followed the school bus all the way to school. He had to be locked up in a room till Sara's mother came to take him home.

Now Chipsie realised why Ann always sent her away as soon as the school bus came. Ann did not want her to follow the school bus and get locked up at school. It was because Ann cared for her that she sent her away from the bus stop every morning.

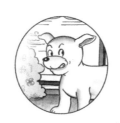

The Dog and the Monkey

A dog used to sit outside a bakery. He would laze around, looking at the people hurrying about with their shopping.

Once, a monkey was waiting for a chance to steal some cupcakes. While the shopkeeper was weighing chocolate chip cookies for a little boy,

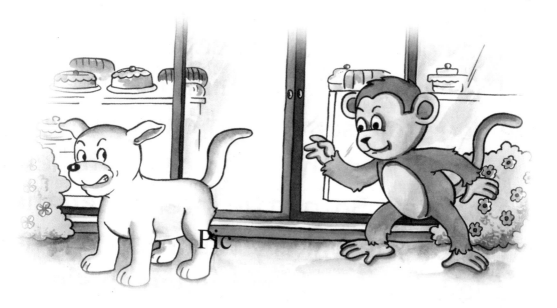

the monkey tried to grab something to eat. But the dog barked and chased away the monkey. The shopkeeper gave the dog a juicy bone as a reward.

There was a meat shop close by. One day, the dog wanted to have some meat. But when he went near the shop, the owner chased him away with a stick.

When the monkey saw this, he told the dog that he would distract the shopkeeper by jumping on his roof and screeching. At that very time the dog could steal some meat.

The monkey started making a noise on the roof. The shopkeeper came out and threw a stick at him. Meanwhile, the dog stole some meat and ran away.

Now it was the dog's turn to help the monkey. So, a little later, when the owner of the bakery was resting, the dog lay down and pretended to sleep.

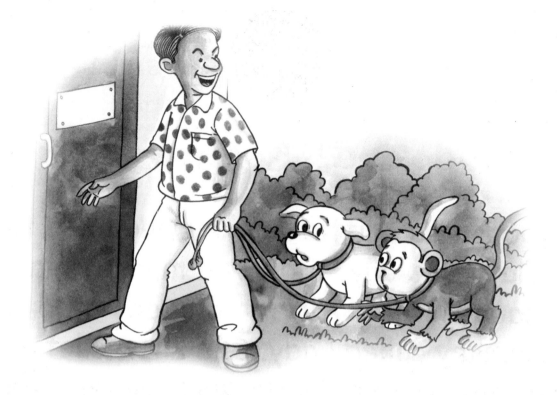

The monkey went in and took some cupcakes.

When the bakery and the meat shop owners understood what the dog and the monkey were up to, they called the stray animal catchers. They were taken to an animal shelter. Here they were served tasteless food. Then they realised they should not have been dishonest.

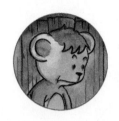

Dodo and the Monkey Man

Dodo was a little monkey who liked to play. One day, Albert, a monkey man, caught him. Albert already had a monkey called Lady. She knew a lot of funny tricks. Dodo was clever and learnt those tricks very fast.

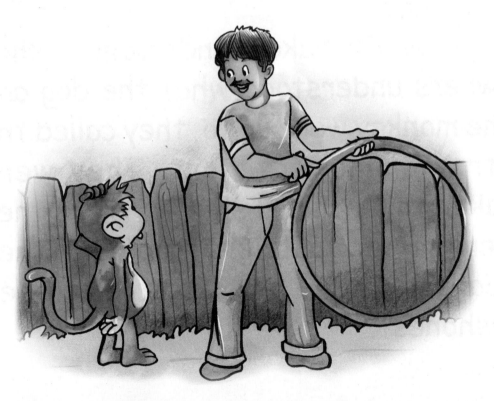

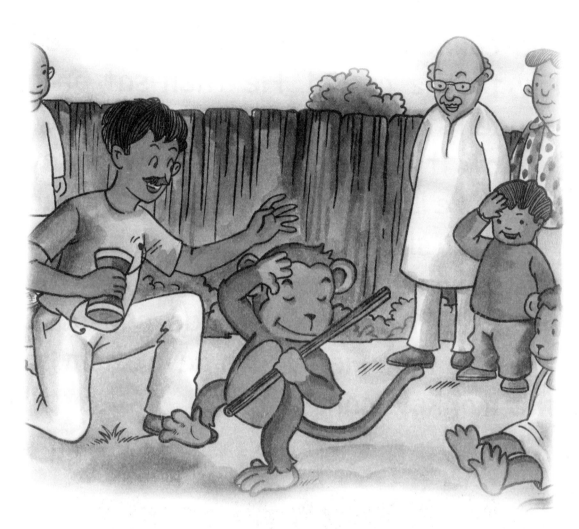

Albert would go from house to house and when a group of children gathered together, he would show them tricks. That would make the children laugh.

One day, after a large group of people had collected around them, the monkey man tugged at Dodo's string and called him forward. Dodo bowed low to the crowd. He then sat on a wooden stool and looked towards Lady.

Now it was her turn. The monkey man gave Lady a small purse. He asked her to go shopping. She picked up some things which Albert had placed on the ground. She went to Dodo and gave them to him. He in turn gave them to the monkey man.

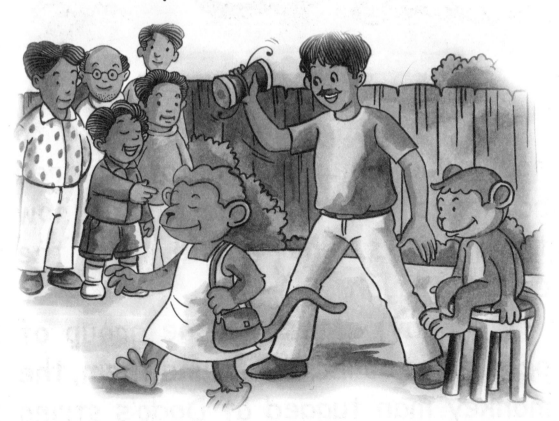

One day, Albert taught Dodo to march like a soldier. Dodo took a stick with a rope and put it across his shoulder like a gun. He marched up and down with Lady and saluted the children. They all clapped for him.

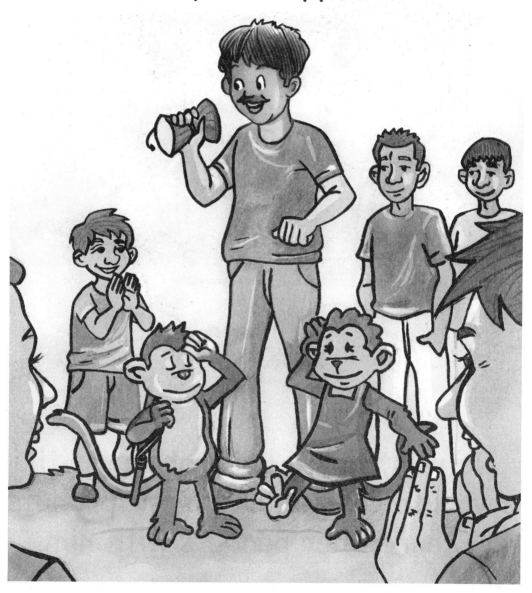

After every show, Albert gave the monkeys some peanuts to eat. One day, he forgot to give some to Dodo. That upset Dodo.

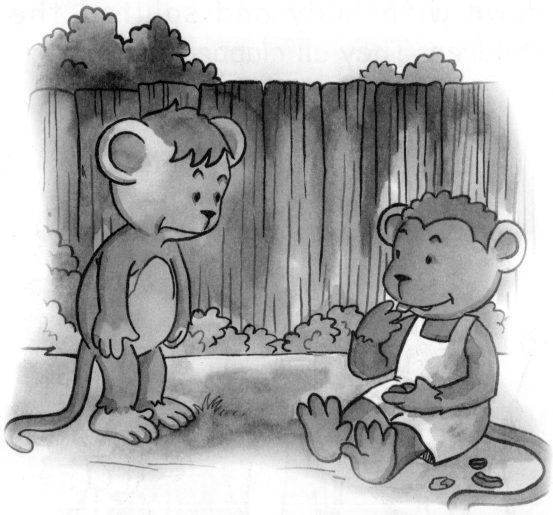

He went up to Lady and said that he would also like to eat some peanuts. Lady shared her peanuts with him.

Once the monkey man dressed Lady in a beautiful white dress and a veil. He made Dodo wear a smart jacket. He was getting them married. The bride acted shy. But Dodo held his head high.

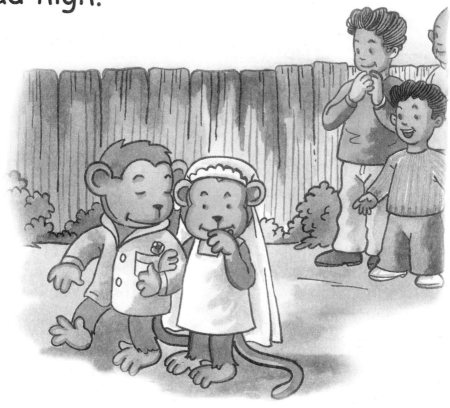

The children were excited. They threw peanuts and popcorn and coins on the married couple. The show ended happily!

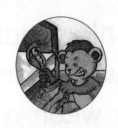

Rambo Saves the Baby

Rambo lived on a tree near Monica's house. He ate fruits from the tree. Monica also got him food from her kitchen. He was a happy monkey.

Rambo used to watch Monica's baby brother, Bobby, through the window. Rambo was very fond of children. So when Monica took the baby for a ride in his pram, Rambo would

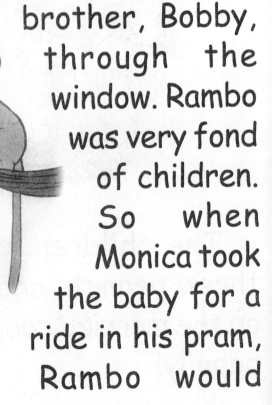

follow them. Sometimes he would sit on a branch outside the window and watch little Bobby sleep. Whenever the baby saw him, he would start clapping his hands.

One day, Rambo was looking at Bobby from his usual place. Suddenly, he saw a small snake enter the room and move towards the baby's bed.

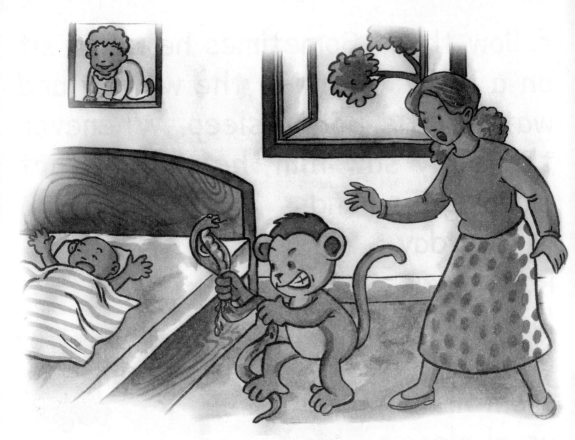

At once, Rambo climbed down from the tree and ran to the house. He jumped into the room and caught the snake. Just then Bobby woke up and started crying.

On hearing Bobby cry, the children's mother came running into the room. She was shocked to see Rambo holding a snake. She screamed in fear. Rambo jumped on to the

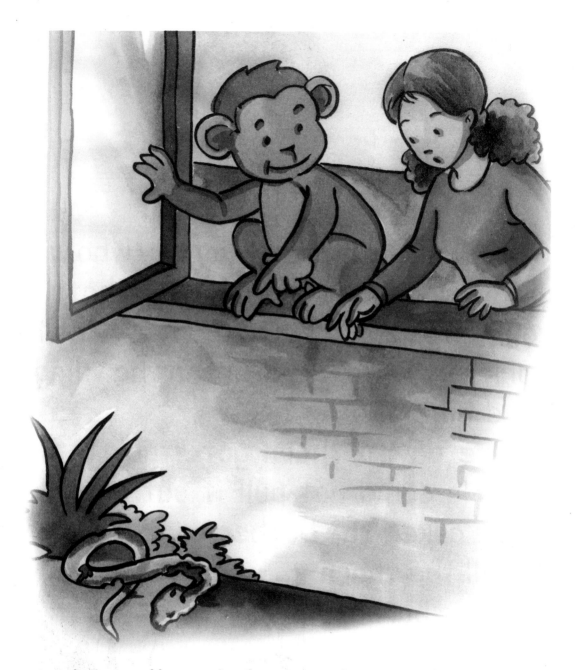

window sill and threw the snake down. He then went back to his branch.

From that day, Rambo became a part of Monica's family.

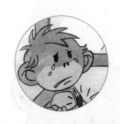

The Lazy Monkey

Once there was a lazy monkey who was always looking for anything that he could get for free. He did not want to work for his food. No one in the village liked him.

One day, a thorn got stuck in his tail. He could not pull it out himself. So he asked the barber to pull the thorn out. The barber was in a hurry. He got the thorn out with his

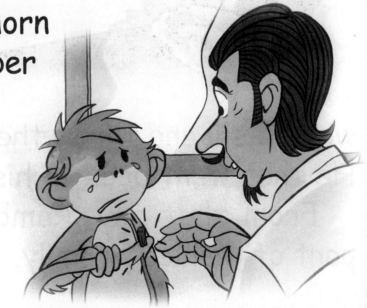

razor, but a little bit of the monkey's tail got cut.

The monkey was very angry.

"Put back my tail or give me your razor!" he said.

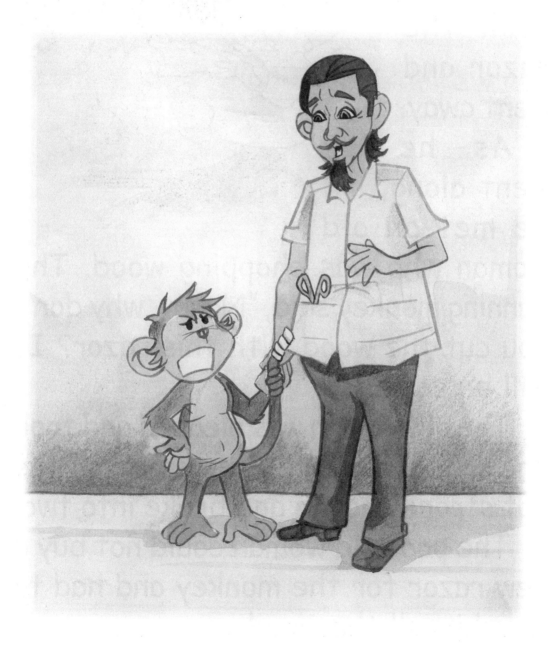

The poor barber had to hand over his razor. The monkey took the razor and went away.

As he went along, he met an old woman who was chopping wood. The cunning monkey said, "Nanny, why don't you cut the wood with this razor? It will be easier."

The old woman was pleased and took the razor from him. But the razor was not strong enough and broke into two.

The poor old woman could not buy a new razor for the monkey and had to give him all the wood.

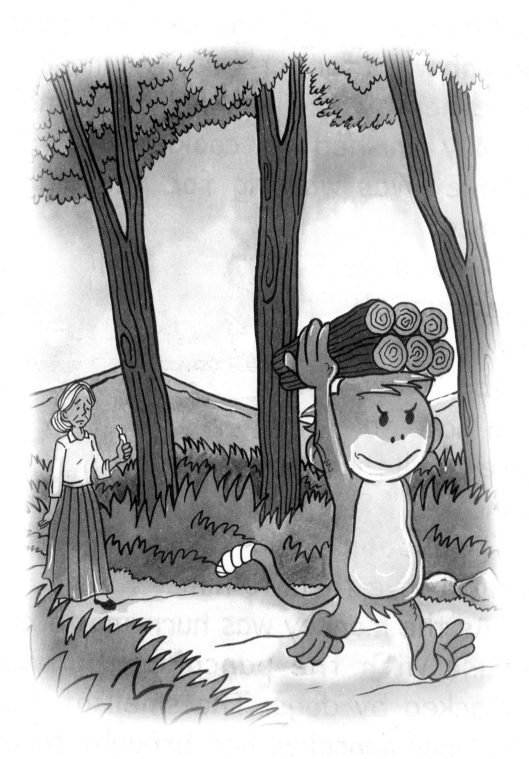

Soon the monkey saw a woman making pancakes. She did not have enough wood for the fire. The monkey gave her all the wood. The woman happily finished her cooking. But the monkey was waiting for the right chance.

"You have used up all my wood," he said. "Now you have to give me all the pancakes!"

The poor woman gave them to him.

As the monkey was hurrying to his house with the pancakes, he was attacked by dogs. The smell of the delicious pancakes had brought them there.

The monkey had to leave the pancakes. He climbed a nearby tree, and unhappily watched the dogs enjoying the pancakes to the last bit.

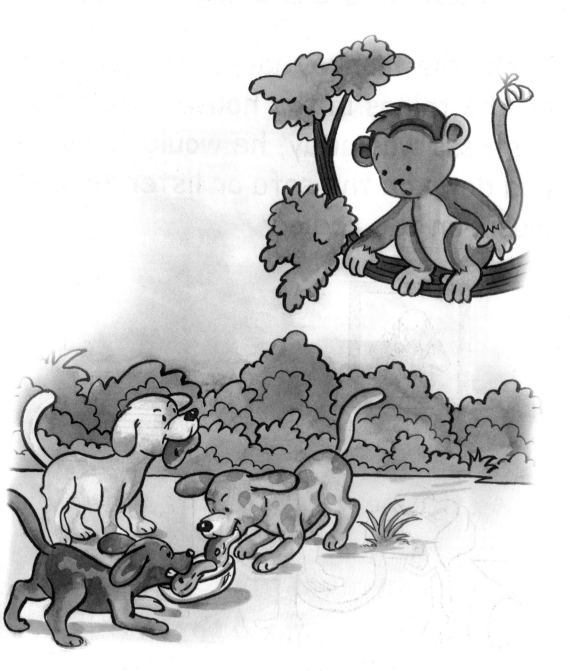

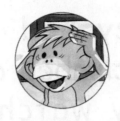

Tashi the Curious Monkey

Tashi the monkey loved to play with all the things in the house. When the mistress was away, he would jump up and down on the sofa or listen to loud music on the radio.

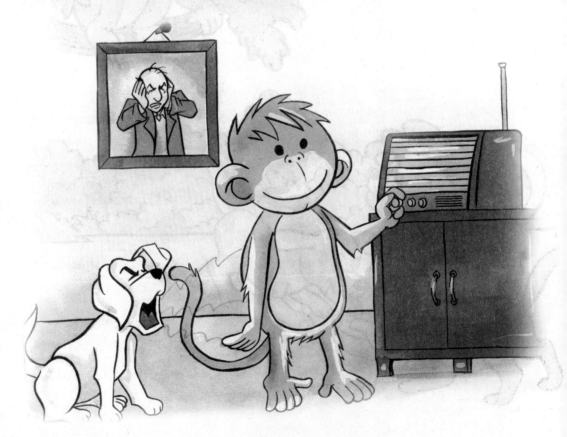

One day, he saw the cassette player and very soon he learnt how to switch it on. He turned up the volume and listened to the music. Tashi then took the cassette player near the window to make the birds hear the music.

"We sing so well ourselves. Why should we listen to your silly music?" they said to him.

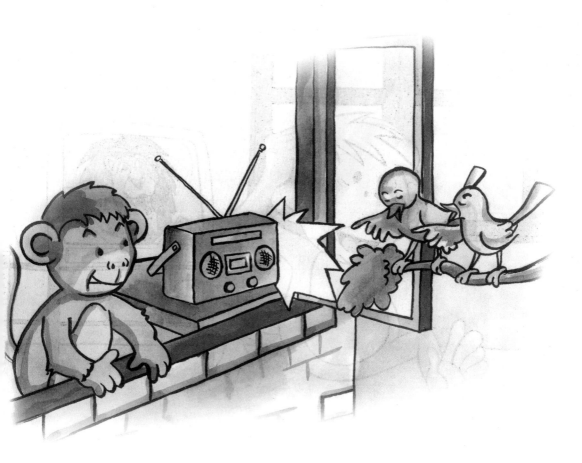

Curious Tashi then decided to fiddle with the knobs of the television set. Suddenly the television switched on. A lion was roaring on the screen and Tashi got scared.

"It is only a picture," the television laughed at Tashi. But Tashi was too scared to go near it again.

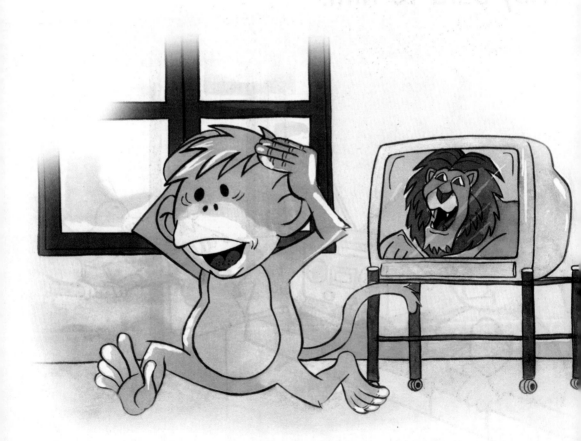

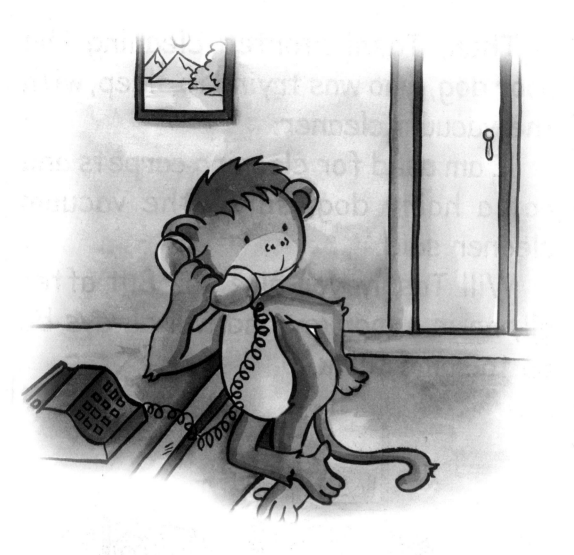

Just then, the telephone rang. Tashi picked it up. Someone spoke at the other end. All Tashi could do was make monkey sounds.

"The telephone is for human beings and not for a silly thing like you," the telephone said.

Then, Tashi started cleaning the poor dog, who was trying to sleep, with the vacuum cleaner.

"I am used for cleaning carpets and not a hairy dog, silly," the vacuum cleaner said.

Will Tashi ever give up? But after all, he is a monkey and will always be up to some trick.

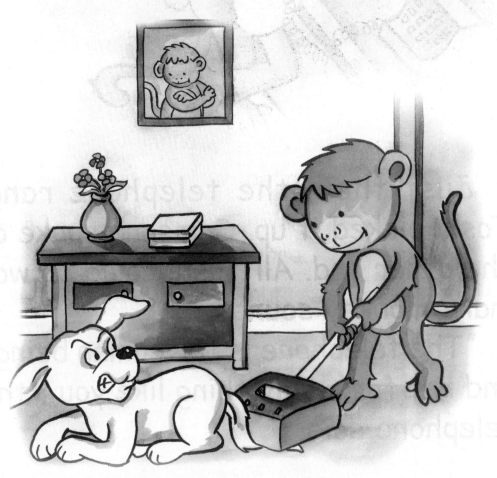

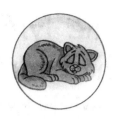

Pandora Finds a Home

I am Pandora. And this is my story.

One early morning my mother left me alone to go in search of food. I waited and waited, but she did not return. I could not go looking for her because I could not even open my eyes. I felt very lost and alone.

Suddenly I felt someone lift me gently. It was a little girl called Nikita.

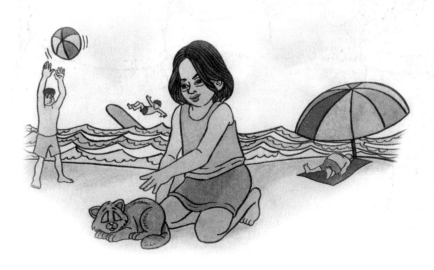

She had seen me lying on the sand while going to the beach. She was on a seaside holiday with her parents. She took me to their hotel.

"I found this little kitten on the beach," Nikita told her mother. "Mummy, please, please, may we keep her?"

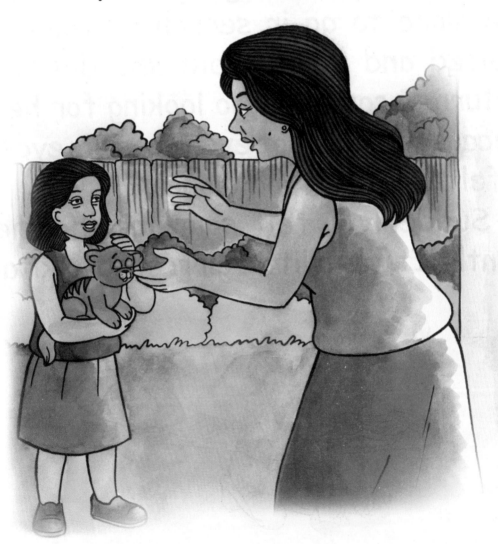

Nikita's mother also loved animals.

"But how will we take her home?" she asked.

"We can take her in a box," Nikita said.

"All right!" said her mother.

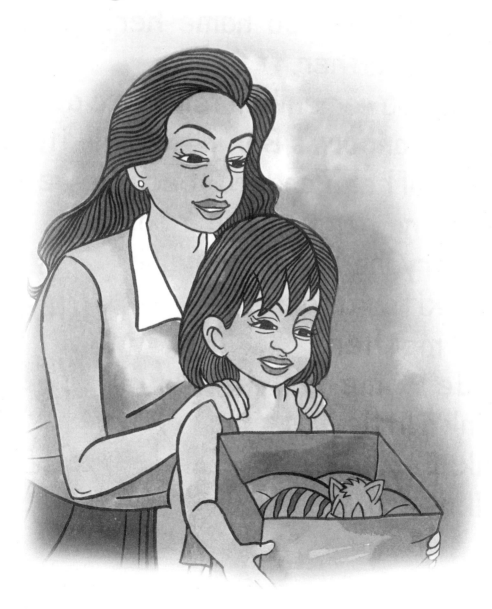

"She seems to be hungry," said Nikita's father. "Let us get her some milk. We will need a dropper to feed her."

He went to the chemist to get a dropper.

"What will you name her?" asked Nikita's mother.

"Do you remember telling me a story called 'Pandora's Box'?" said Nikita. "I shall call her 'Pandora', because we will be taking her home in a box!"

Everyone liked the name.

Nikita and her mother made me drink a little milk. I soon fell asleep.

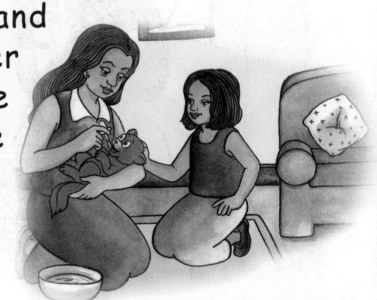

But every now and then, I would mew and turn a bit. Then Nikita covered me with a scarf and I became comfortable.

In the car, Nikita kept me in the box on her lap. Once in a while, she would check on me and feed me milk.

We were home by the evening. Nikita made a special corner for me in her room. She fed me milk every day.

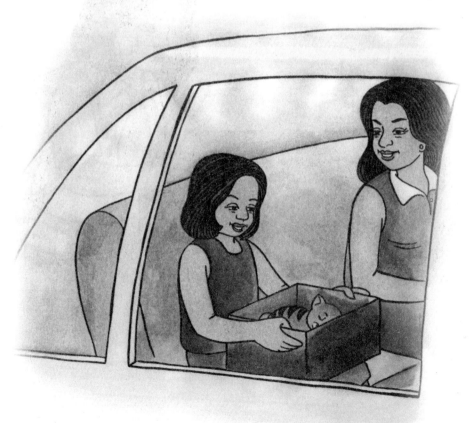

Soon it was time for Nikita to go back to school. But the moment she returned home from school every day, she would rush to meet me.

In a few days I began to move about in the box. When I was taken out, I would mew and try to walk. I was happy. I had found a loving home.

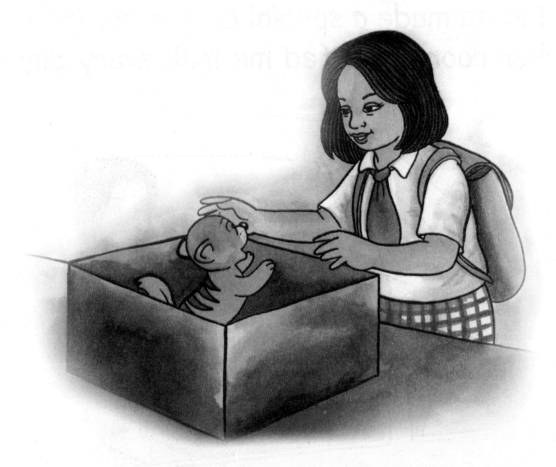

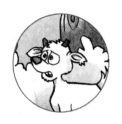

The Clever Goat

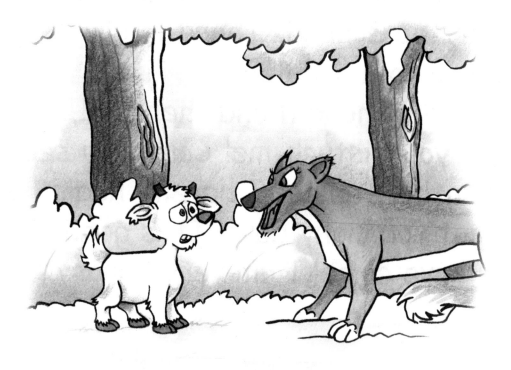

Once a naughty goat fought with her mother and ran away from her. Soon, she was lost in the forest and got scared. She climbed a hill to look for the rest of the herd. Suddenly, she saw a jackal looking greedily at her.

"Oh my pretty sister, you look lost. Come with me, I will show you the way to your herd," he said.

The goat was very frightened, but she remembered her mother's words, "Don't be scared. There is always an answer to a problem."

So she thought and then said, "How dare you disturb me! Can't you see I am eating stones? I haven't had a lion to eat for many days! It is good that you have come! I am very hungry."

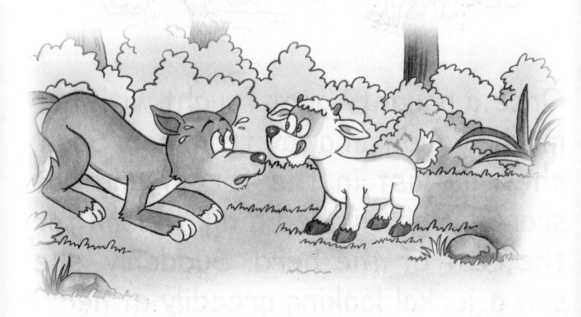

The jackal thought that she was a witch in the form of a goat and would kill him for food. So he ran away as fast as he could.

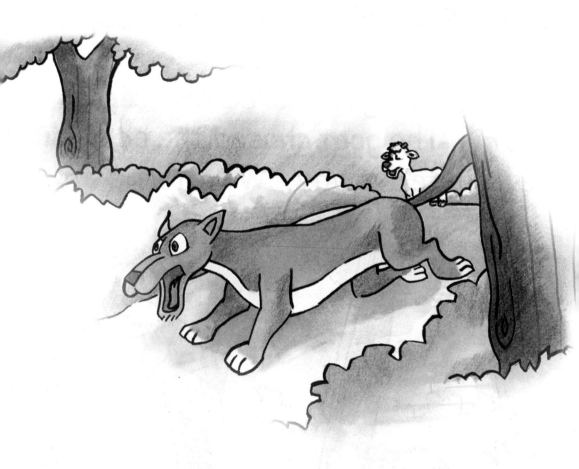

Just then, the goat saw a bear running towards her. She had to think of something fast.

"Hurry up, you dirty thing! Why didn't you come sooner? I am dying of hunger. A whole jackal was not enough. I need a couple of lions to fill my stomach. But for now, you will do," she said loudly.

The bear got scared and ran down the hill. The goat chased the bear, but he slipped away. When the goat

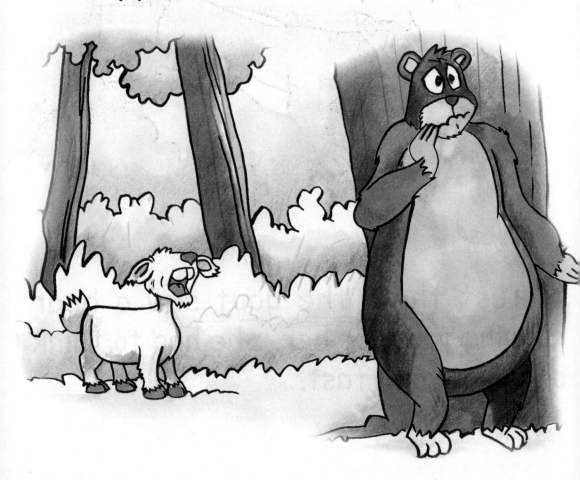

stopped, she saw that she had come out of the forest. She saw her mother with the rest of the herd and ran to join them.

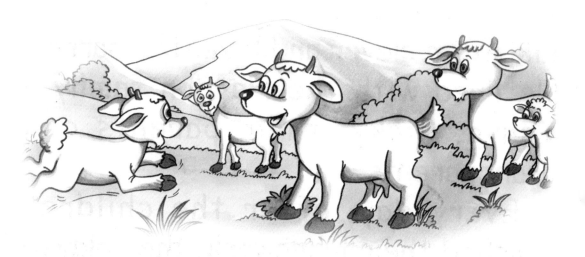

"Where did you go?" said her mother. "We were looking everywhere for you."

The goat told her mother about her adventures. Her mother laughed and said, "You have been very brave and clever. But don't run away like this again. Next time you may not be so lucky!"

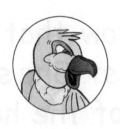

Kiki the Parrot

Kiki was a clever and beautiful parrot. He lived with the Haydon family – Tanya, Ricky, their parents and grandparents.

Every day, after the children finished their homework, they played and talked to Kiki. They had taught him many words.

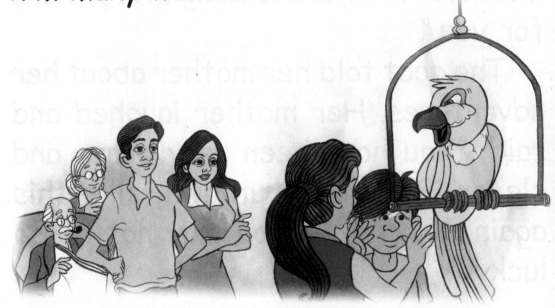

In the morning, Kiki said, "Good morning." When he was given peanuts or green chillies or a guava, he would say, "Thank you." When the children went to school, Kiki would say, "Bye Bye!" If someone entered the room, Kiki would ask, "Who is there?"

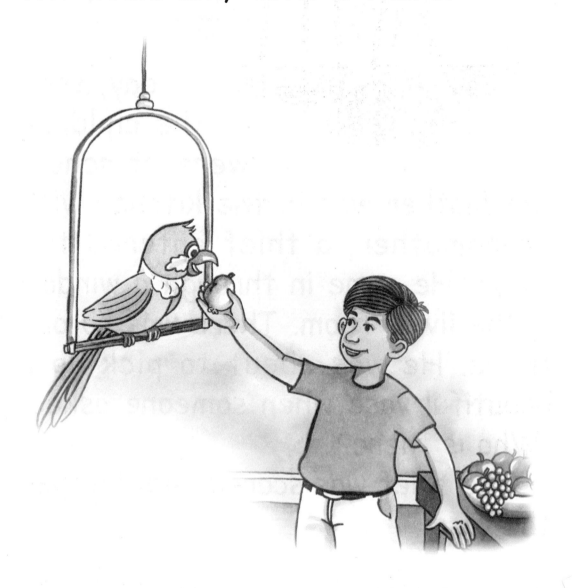

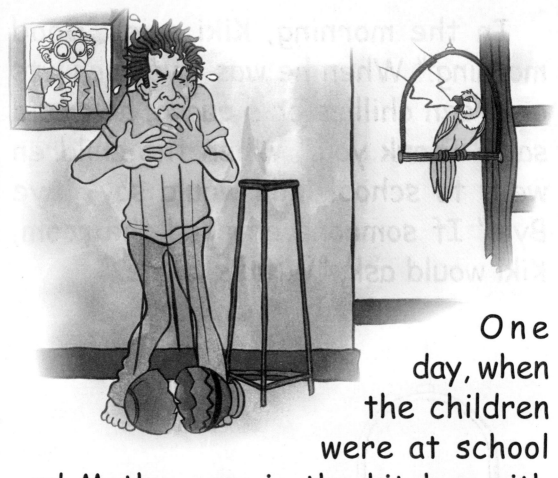

One day, when the children were at school and Mother was in the kitchen with Grandmother, a thief entered the house. He came in through a window in the living room. There was no one there. He was about to pick up a beautiful vase when someone asked, "Who is there?"

The thief was scared and dropped the vase.

Kiki had asked the question! The thief thought there was someone in the room. He rushed out of the house.

Mother heard the crash and came to the living room. When she saw a young man running out of the gate, she shouted, "Thief, thief! Help!" But the thief ran away. Mother realised that the thief must have heard Kiki talking.

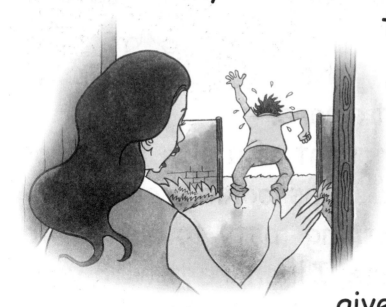

That evening, Kiki was given a special treat of his favourite fruits and peanuts. Kiki's day was made!

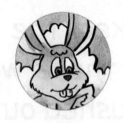

The Tiger and the Hare

Once, far away in a jungle, there lived a cruel tiger.

One day, the tiger caught a hare. The hare thought of a plan to escape.

"Oh Lord! I was looking for you. I've found something tasty to eat. If you come with me, I'll share it with you."

The tiger wanted to try the tasty food. He went with the hare deeper into the jungle. Soon, they reached a heap of eleven smooth, white stones. The hare picked up one and said, "Here it is. Once you've eaten these, you'll never like anything else."

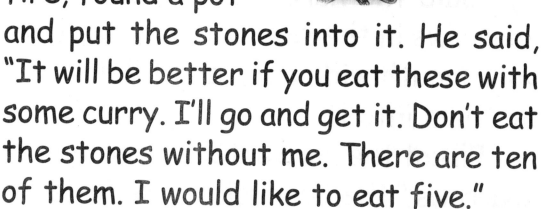

The hare lit a fire, found a pot and put the stones into it. He said, "It will be better if you eat these with some curry. I'll go and get it. Don't eat the stones without me. There are ten of them. I would like to eat five."

The tiger counted the stones, and found that there were eleven of them.

"If I eat one, it won't be missed," he thought. He greedily picked up one and tossed it into his mouth. He yelled and howled with pain as the burning hot stone went down his throat and into his stomach. The clever hare watched the fun from behind a bush.

A few days later, the tiger saw the hare and caught him.

"This time you can't fool me, you cunning hare!" he said.

"Oh! I was hoping you would come by," said the hare. "Do you see those sparrows in the sky? Just look up with your mouth wide open and I'll drive all of them into it."

"I'll eat the hare after I've eaten the sparrows," the tiger told himself. He sat with his mouth open, looking upwards.

The hare lit a fire around the tiger and ran away.

The tiger suddenly saw to his horror that there was fire all around him. He burnt himself while trying to escape. He was angry because he had been fooled by the hare once again.

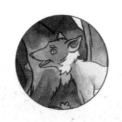

The Clever Fox

One day, a lion saw a fox eating honey from his tree! He told him to get down at once.

The cunning fox leaped down and ran into the jungle before the lion could catch him.

The lion then went looking for the fox, but his lair was empty. So the lion waited for the fox inside his lair.

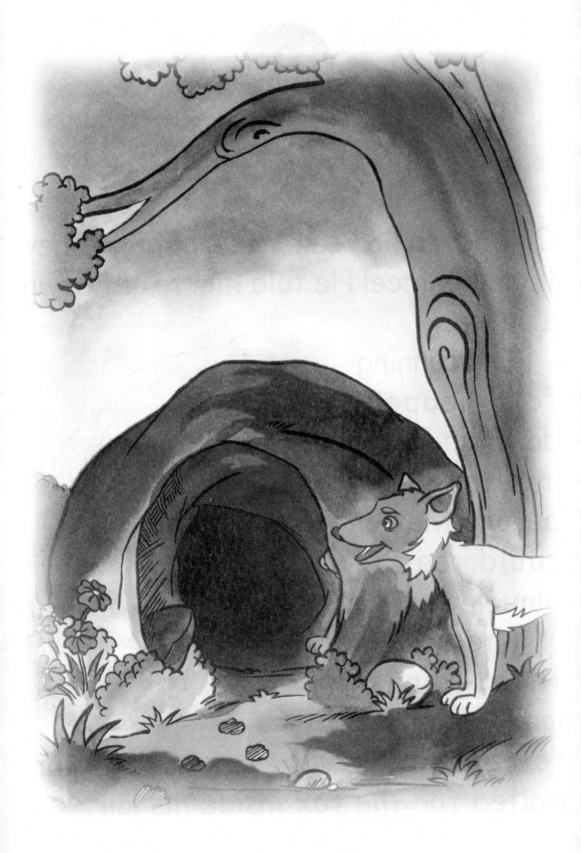

Soon the fox came home. He saw the footprints of the lion going into his lair. He understood that the lion was lying in wait for him inside. He shouted, "Good day, my dear house. It's good to be home again."

When he got no reply, the fox again said, "Good day, my dear house. Why don't you talk to me? You always do so every day when I come home."

The lion thought for a while and said, "Good day. Welcome home."

The fox laughed aloud and said, "Oh, you stupid lion! Have you ever heard a house talking? I know for sure now, that you are hiding inside. Now you can't get me."

The lion ran out to catch him, but the fox was, once again, too quick for him.

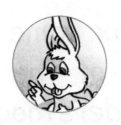

The brave hare

Once upon a time, a small hare lived in a jungle. He was called Long Tail, because of his long bushy tail. He got scared very easily, but he wanted to become brave.

One day, Long Tail was boasting to a group of hares, "I am not afraid of

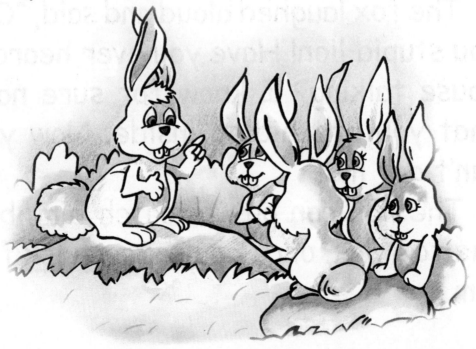

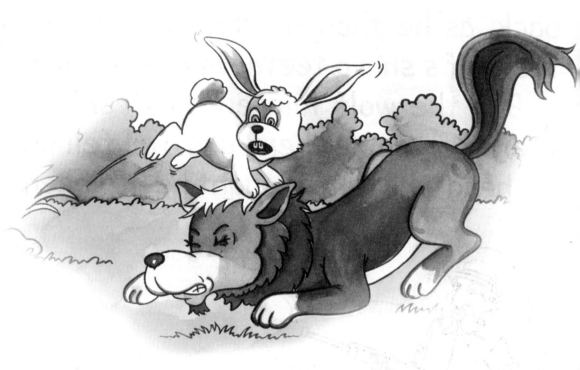

anyone – not the tiger, nor the bear. In fact, if I see a wolf, I will eat it up."

Just as he finished speaking, he saw a hungry wolf staring at him. The wolf was about to jump on him. Long Tail was so scared that he jumped and landed on the wolf's head, rolled off his back, and ran as fast as he could, deep into the woods.

Long Tail kept running till he could run no more. He did not turn to look back, as he thought that any minute the wolf's sharp teeth would bite him.

But the wolf himself was running the other way. When Long Tail fell on his head, the wolf thought he had been

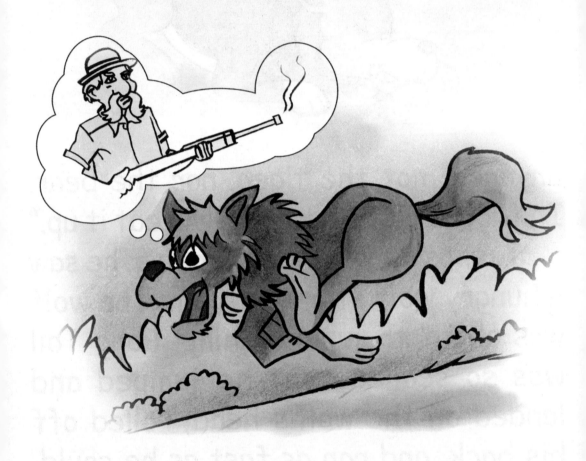

hit by a hunter's bullet. Without stopping to see what had happened, he had started running.

The other hares had hidden wherever they could – behind bushes or in hollow trunks.

Later, the braver hares peeped out of their holes and then stepped out. The others followed.

"Long Tail has really chased the wolf away," said an old, wise hare.

"Yes. Otherwise, we would not have been alive just now," said another.

"But where is Long Tail?" asked the others.

They all started looking for him. After a long time, they found him in a hole, shaking with fear.

"Bravo, Long Tail! You are a hero," they all shouted. "You chased the wolf away. Thank you so much! All this time we thought that you were boasting. But you really are brave!"

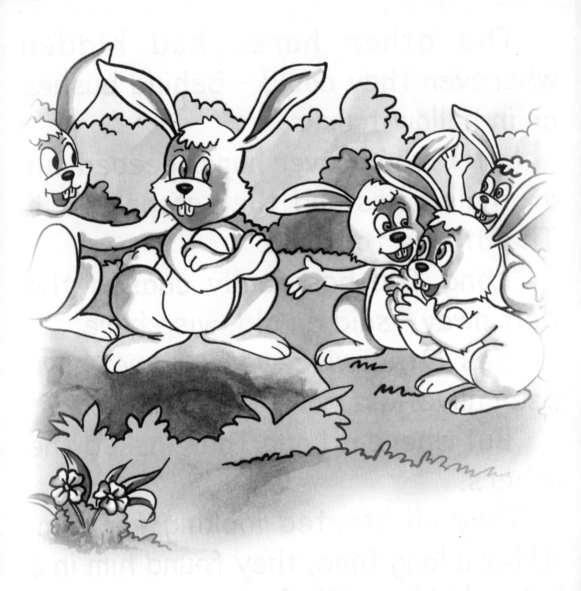

Long Tail was surprised to hear the other hares praise him.

From that day onwards, Long Tail really thought himself to be a brave little hare!

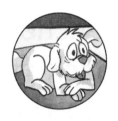

Patch Finds a Home

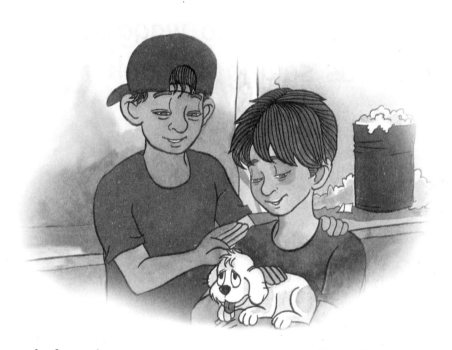

A sad-looking pup sat near a pile of garbage at the corner of the street. Aaron and Sunny were walking past him when they heard him whining. Sunny picked up the lost pup. The boys felt sorry for him. They decided to take him home.

When they reached home, Father had also come back from work. They showed the pup to their parents. The brothers wanted to keep him. They jumped with joy when their parents agreed. The pup too wagged his tail, as if he was saying, "Thank you."

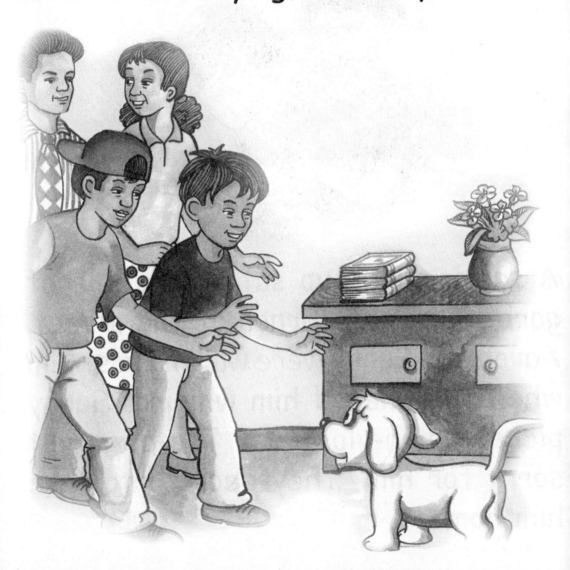

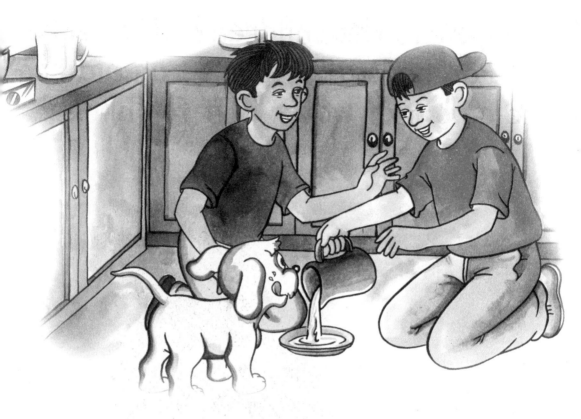

They took him to the kitchen and poured some warm milk in a saucer for him. He lapped it up hungrily. Everyone started thinking of names for the pup. By the time they decided on the name 'Patch', the little pup had already gone to sleep!

Everyone at home loved Patch. He would sit quietly at Grandmother's feet every morning while she read the newspaper. The children built a kennel for Patch. Mother placed an old rug and a bowl of water in it for him.

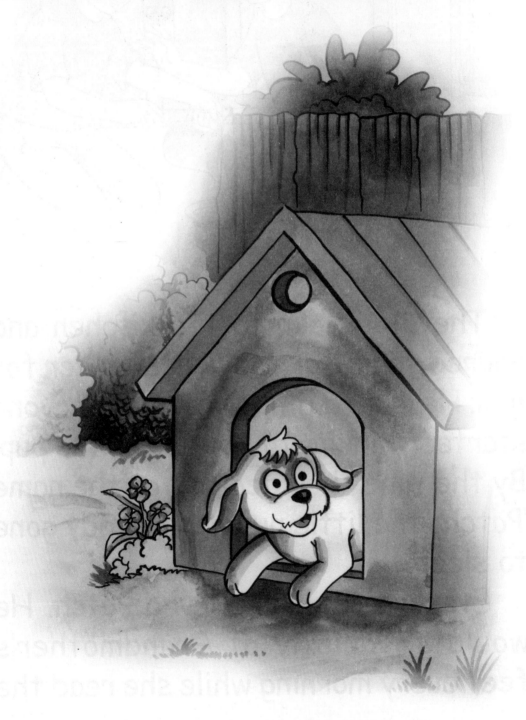

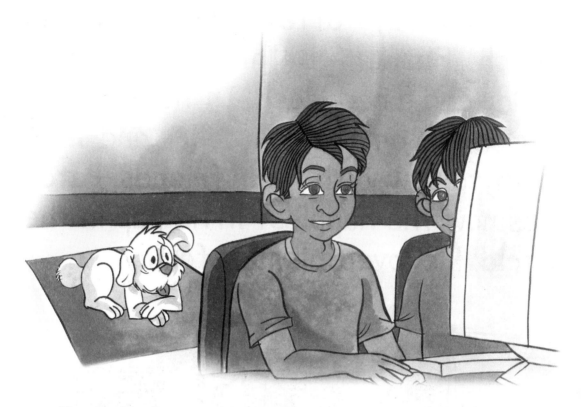

Patch loved waiting for Aaron and Sunny to come home from school. As soon as they got off their school bus, he would rush to them. After that, he followed them all day till they got into bed. He went to the park and played with their friends. When the boys sat at their computer, he sat on the rug nearby, staring at the screen – as if he understood everything!

A few days after they had found Patch, Father got him a shiny red collar and a red leash. In the evening, Aaron put on the new collar and they went to play with their friends. Patch was now the happiest little pup in the world. He loved his new family.

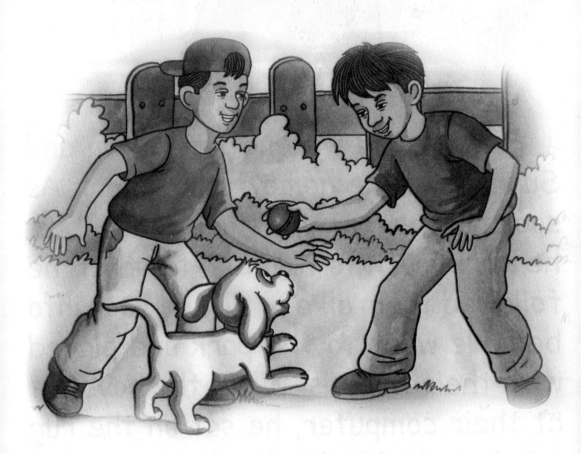

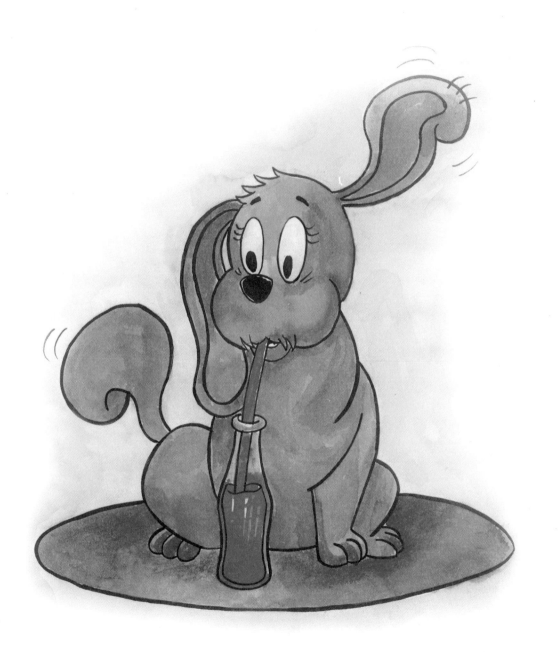